About the Author
Eli Ginzberg is Director of the Conservation of Human Resources Project, Columbia University. He is also the author of *The Coming Physician Surplus* (with Miriam Ostow; Rowman & Allanheld 1984).

American Medicine: The Power Shift

American Medicine

THE POWER SHIFT

Eli Ginzberg

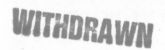

ROWMAN & ALLANHELD
PUBLISHERS

ROWMAN & ALLANHELD

Published in the United States of America in 1985
by Rowman & Allanheld, Publishers
(a division of Littlefield, Adams & Company)
81 Adams Drive, Totowa, New Jersey 07512

Library of Congress Cataloging in Publication Data

Ginzberg, Eli, 1911-
  American medicine.

  Bibliography: p. 194
  Includes index.
  1. Medical economics—United States.   2. Medical care
—United States.   3. Medical personnel—United States.
I. Title. [DNLM: 1. Cost Control—trends—United States.
2. Delivery of Health Care—economics—United States.
3. Economics, Medical—trends—United States. W 74 G493a]
RA410.53.G56   1985   362.1'0973   85-8173
ISBN 0-8476-7439-8

85 86 87 / 10 9 8 7 6 5 4 3 2 1
Printed in the United States of America

To Miriam and Mortimer Ostow,
for a friendship of four decades

Contents

Preface

This book contains the most important efforts I made in the early 1980s to understand the unsolved problems facing the U.S. health care system and to identify the preferred solutions. There is little point in our seeking ways to constrain the continuing increases in health care costs if in the process we hobble medical innovation, place new barriers in the path of the elderly and the poor who need access to the system, and so bind the practice of medicine with rules and regulations that physicians become disenchanted with their profession and their work. My intention has been to illuminate for the reader the complex and subtle trade-offs that are required if U.S. medical care is to continue in the vanguard and still remain affordable.

Acknowledgment is made to The Robert Wood Johnson Foundation, the Commonwealth Fund, and the Health Services Foundation, a research affiliate of the Blue Cross and Blue Shield Association, whose research support during the first half of the 1980s facilitated the preparation of these essays.

Mrs. Miriam Ostow, my senior associate in our health studies program at the Conservation of Human Resources Project, Columbia University, has contributed a great deal to sharpening the arguments and to refining the analyses, for which I am greatly in her debt.

My wife, Ruth S. Ginzberg, has once again used her light editorial pencil to smooth the text, for which the reader and I are in her debt.

Ms. Shoshana Vasheetz and Mr. Patrick Muldowney carried out the task of preparing the manuscript for the publisher, an undertaking for which I am grateful.

Eli Ginzberg
April 1985

Foreword

Progress and Problems

When our expenditures for health care in 1984 become known we will probably learn that the United States spent close to $400 billion for its health care, about 11 percent of the Gross National Product (GNP). This means that expenditures for health care approximate those for food or housing and are three times as large as the amounts the American public spends on clothing.

Another comparison can be made between the total outlays for health and the expenditures of the federal government. The nation spent considerably more on health than the federal government did on defense. Total national outlays for health were approximately equal to all federal expenditures for human resources—social security (less health), veterans, and education and training.

There is no way to reach a judgment about the amount of money that individuals and nations should devote to the purchase of specific goods and services. In fact, these decisions result from the joint decisions reached by the citizenry about how to allocate its earnings, less the amount that it is willing to pay in taxes, which in turn are spent by politicians who listen to the preferences of their constituents.

Some clues to spending behavior can be extracted by making comparisons with times past, by looking at the patterns of other advanced societies, and in considering information gained from opinion surveys. Using these criteria, we have reached the following conclusions: Since the end of World War II the United States has more than tripled the proportion of the GNP that it devotes to health care, from about 3.5 to 11 percent. In terms of constant dollars from which the inflation factor has been extracted and which has taken population growth into consideration, the expenditures per capita for health care have grown by a factor of 10 in the half century between the administrations of President Hoover and President Reagan.

When we look at comparative data across national borders, we find that, on a per capita basis, the United Kingdom spends much less, Canada somewhat less, and Germany, Sweden, and the Netherlands in the same range as the United States—circa 10 to 11 percent of GNP.

Finally, repeated opinion surveys in this country reveal a growing consensus among most groups that the costs of medical care are too high in that we are not getting fair value for our money. Waste in the system is grounded in such diverse forces as excessive use by consumers who are covered by insurance; inefficiencies in hospital operations, which reflect the fact that most hospitals have been reimbursed for their costs or charges; excessive earnings by physicians who have been protected from having to compete with each other on the basis of price; and the additional costs that result from the heavy hand of federal and state regulators.

This growing concern with our steeply rising health care costs is not new, although it has become more pervasive of late. And it does not provide a balanced view of how the American people feel about their health care system. The same opinion surveys that report on a growing restiveness about the acceleration of costs also provide information that points to the broad satisfaction of the public with access to providers and with the quality of care that they receive. In fact, on balance, the public favors an expansion of the system and looks favorably on increasing the range and quality of the available health services, without specifying how the additional services should be paid for, and by whom.

One way to understand the progress that has been made to obtain insight into the problems that lie ahead is to look more closely at the transformations that have been underway since the end of World War II, that is, to focus on changes during the last two generations. A relatively small number of developments can explain the major expansion of the system.

First, medicine was in a good position to make major advances on a series of fronts—diagnostic, therapeutic, and rehabilitative. Victory over most of the infectious diseases had recently been achieved. The great postwar triumph was the ability to protect the entire population against poliomyelitis. The elements that had been responsible for previous major advances consisted of new biomedical knowledge and new techniques, the education and training of larger numbers of physicians and supporting personnel, and a sufficient inflow of dollars to provide the capital and operating funds required to assure access for most of the population to these services.

Three developments were responsible for the structure of the health care system in the United States prior to the war's outbreak. At that time, American medicine still looked to Europe for most advances in knowledge and for many advances in technique. Young American physicians preparing for a career in a specialty usually arranged to spend a postgraduate year or two in Germany or Austria, until Hitler laid his heavy hand on university and research establishments.

The U.S. medical educational establishment was tightly controlled by leadership who sought to keep the total numbers of students in balance with the ability of the marketplace to absorb them when they graduated; it further exercised a selective admissions policy that was strongly prejudiced against women, certain ethnic groups, and non-Protestants.

Third, the economic foundation of the health care system had serious weaknesses. Roosevelt had decided against including health care coverage in his Social Security legislation of 1935. Nongovernment insurance for hospital and other high-cost health care services was still in an embryonic stage; many communities had neither a hospital nor a physician; many persons with limited incomes had to depend on philanthropy or underfunded government institutions even for emergency care. Most of the blacks in the South, about 80 percent of all blacks, had restricted access to the system.

These characteristics of the system provide perspective on the progress that has been achieved since the end of World War II as well as on the problems that confront the system in 1985. The current litany of complaints and concerns include a belief that medical knowledge and technique are advancing at too rapid a rate, as evidenced by the purchase of ever more costly equipment by hospitals and physicians and the certification of more and more specialists and subspecialists who greatly exceed the number that informed observers believe are required to provide a superior level of care. The educational-research base is considered by many to be seriously distorted. The conclusion of the prestigious Graduate Medical Education National Advisory Committee (GMENAC) (1980) is that by 1990, the United States will face a surplus of more than 70,000 physicians, and by century's end a surplus of more than 140,000.

The situation on the research front is not as clear. If we knew how to translate more dollar expenditures into more useful knowledge, as was the anticipation of President Nixon and the Congress in 1970 when they enlarged the appropriations for the National Cancer Institute, the country would even now be willing to expand its biomedical research base. But since more dollars do not translate immediately or within a real time frame into additional useful knowledge, the federal government and the private sector have decided to proceed at a more measured pace. Further, government, industry, and the medical profession are giving serious consideration to regulating the rate at which new medical technology is introduced, a move dictated both by a desire to contain total expenditures and to provide time to assess prospective innovations.

As noted above, there were deficiencies in the health care system at the war's end: not only was there a shortage in many areas of properly equipped and staffed hospitals, but the United States also lacked a financing mechanism that would enable its citizens to meet the costs of a major illness without beggaring themselves. In 1985, many leaders of opinion believe that the primary reason for our health care costs being out of control is that insurance and government entitlement programs have provided so much money that the consumer no longer exercises any constraint when seeking medical care.

How can we explain the past four decades of major changes that eliminated deficiencies in our health care system? These changes included a marked expansion and improvement in the educational-research base, a major inflow of new resources to provide a greatly expanded infrastructure for health care delivery, and the implementation of broad-based financing that assures easy access for most of the population to acute hospitals and to many other important health care services. The answer to this rhetorical question will provide better understanding of our progress as well as the reasons why we still face a host of unsolved problems.

In broad strokes, the answers follow. One of the lasting impacts of the war was the knowledge gained by public and private sector alike that research and development are important. In the intervening four decades we increased our total annual outlays for medical research from around $150 million to about $10 billion; most of the expansion occurred prior to 1970, with the level in constant dollars maintained thereafter.

Medical education had been under the control of the medical establishment since the Flexner Report was released (1910), and most costs were covered by state governments or philanthropy. In the early postwar period when patients had to wait to see their physicians, the federal government offered to help expand the educational base; but the AMA declined the offer. Its veto held until 1963, when it decided to use its influence to defeat Medicare. After both the state and federal governments appropriated large sums to expand admissions to medical schools, annual enrollments and graduates doubled. With a big boost from the inflow of foreign medical graduates, the ratio of physicians per 100,000 population increased from 140 in 1950 to 210 in 1983; it will reach 240 by this decade's end and 280 by the year 2000, when it will be double the 1950 ratio. Qualitatively the gains will be even greater, because physicians on the average have experienced a doubling in the years of preparation, from five to ten.

Twice during the immediate postwar years President Truman tried to have national health insurance enacted into law, and both times was roundly defeated. The proposal was doomed not only by the violent opposition of the AMA, the insurance industry, corporate leadership, and the voluntary hospital sector, but also by the paucity of support: a few labor leaders, a few medical reformers, a few social welfare proponents. But it was the growth of private insurance (the Blues and commercial carriers), stimulated by the War Labor Board's decision that health care benefits were outside the scope of wage regulations, that proved decisive. Within a decade after the war's end most workers (and their dependents) had hospital insurance.

That left the poor and the elderly at risk. When it became clear to Congress that the complicated alternatives involving federal-state collaborative financing would not be responsive to the need, Medicare and Medicaid were passed by large majorities in 1965. President Johnson, seeking to assuage the anger and hurt of the AMA, promised that the new legislation would leave undisturbed patient-physician relations, which, it must be emphasized, were predicated on fee-for-service medicine.

One additional observation: as early as 1946 Congress had passed the Hill-Burton Act, which facilitated the flow of federal and state funds into communities to help erect or expand their hospital facilities, a critical element in strengthening the health care infrastructure.

The chapters that follow explore the complex forces that played themselves out on each of these major fronts and point up the anticipated, as well as the unanticipated, interactions among them. They help to explain the actions that our society took to expand and improve health care services for the entire population—an effort that achieved marked success—and at the same time it created a host of problems such as excessively sophisticated technology, a surplus of physicians, excess hospital beds, acute financial problems for government and corporations, and accelerating costs. These new problems invite actions that at worst could fail to produce constructive answers while undermining the substantial progress that the nation has achieved. Our medical care system is expensive, but it provides high-quality care for most of our citizens. Our system also provides a wide range of choices, and it continues to encourage the discovery and the application of new knowledge, which alone can assure better outcomes at affordable costs.

PART I

A Tale of Four Decades

The expansion of the health care system since the end of World War II has no precedent; the changes in all their facets have been pervasive and far-reaching. At the war's end, modern medicine was poised for major advances via breakthroughs in antibiotics and advances in surgery, which was followed in time by advances in professional education and training, the vast increase in health resources, and the broadened access of the entire population to the health care system.

The four pieces that comprise Part I will place this major transformation in perspective. As with all issues on the nation's political agenda—and medicine has been there since World War II—ideology and facts are often confused. The protagonists for and the opponents of major changes move back and forth in their arguments between the facts as they are and the facts as they would like them to be. This confusion is most pervasive in the ongoing arguments about the respective roles of the profit sector, the voluntary sector, and government in shaping and reshaping our medical care system. Chapter 1 distinguishes between facts and preferences and postulates that, politics aside, the U.S. health care system has been and continues to be a mixed system, that is, one in which all three sectors—profit, voluntary, and public—play a role and no one sector determines the outcome.

Chapter 2 explains how the role and influence of the philanthropic sector receded as more and more of the population was covered by health insurance, at least for major medical expenditures, in the first two decades after World War II. With the passage of Medicare and Medicaid in 1965, which assured similar coverage for the elderly and the poor, the entire system became monetarized, and the share of government increased from roughly one-quarter to over two-fifths of all expenditures for health care.

The large new funds that entered the health care system with the 1965 legislation accelerated the rapid inflation in health care prices, which exceeded the rise in the consumer price index, with the result that health care commanded a larger share of our ever-larger total national income. Small wonder that legislators and others concerned with health care policy during the recent past have focused on "cost containment." But, as Chapter 3 explains, true cost containment in the sense of fewer inputs used to provide the same quantity and quality of output has been confused with different payers seeking to reduce *their* costs without concern for changes in the total costs or the total output of the system.

The long Chapter 4 focuses on the nature of the health care delivery system during the post-World War II era, assesses how it has changed, and calls attention to the probable directions of future change. It concludes by calling attention to an often-neglected point: While national and state financing and other decision-making centers can influence the structure and functioning of the health care delivery system, in the final analysis the quantity and quality of the health care available will depend on the resources available in each geographic area and on the conditions that govern the access of different groups to these resources. This is true not only for the health care system in the United States, but also for those under the sole direction of national governments, such as in the United Kingdom and the U.S.S.R.

1

Our Private-Public System

A summary consideration of the conditions governing the flow of capital into health care, the education and training of physicians and other health personnel, and the changing contours of the demand for health services should illuminate our central theme—the respective roles of government and the nongovernmental sector since the end of World War II.

With respect to the flow of capital, the federal government assumed a leading role when it passed the Hill-Burton Act in 1946. It is worth noting that the leader of the Republican conservatives, Senator Robert Taft, supported the bill. This new source of governmental funding stimulated the voluntary sector to increase its efforts to raise capital, especially in many small communities that lacked a hospital.

The federal government also took the lead, which the Blues followed, in recognizing depreciation as a proper charge in its reimbursement formula for hospital care. Following the passage of Medicare and Medicaid in 1965, federal depreciation allowances and cost reimbursement created the preconditions for nonprofit hospitals to enter the capital markets and borrow substantial funds for building, renovation, and equipment. Government provided another assist through its authorization of tax-exempt bonds.

Even this abbreviated account of capital flows into health care must not overlook the fact that the federal government, through the National Institutes of Health and other instrumentalities, as well as many state governments, made considerable funds available for capital projects in the field of medical education and research.[1]

Originally published as "The Nature and Interrelationships of the Private and Public Sectors in Health Services," The Michael M. Davis Lecture Series, Center for Health Administration Studies, Graduate School of Business, University of Chicago, 1983. Reprinted by permission.

Finally, all levels of government spent large sums for the erection of new hospitals and the modernization of existing facilities which served patients for whom they had primary responsibility—the military, veterans, the mentally ill, and the indigent in need of acute care.

In sum, government and the voluntary sector provided the overwhelming proportion of new capital which undergirded the rapid expansion of the health care sector, surely up to 1970; without government support via depreciation, cost reimbursement, and tax exemption it is unlikely that nonprofit hospitals would have been able to tap the private capital market in the 1970s and early 1980s.

If one shifts the focus to the education and training of physicians and other health personnel—the foundation of a health care delivery system—one again finds state and federal governments in lead roles with the voluntary sector also an important contributor. Responsibility for the training of physicians had long been divided among state governments, nonprofit universities, and a limited number of freestanding medical schools, a pattern that continued in the postwar period, supplemented by the belated admission to partnership of the federal government.

The years between 1945 and 1960 saw a relatively slow response by the states to the need for new medical schools and the expansion of existing ones. The voluntary sector also moved slowly, primarily because of the high costs that were involved. Congress indicated its willingness to participate in the effort, a policy successfully thwarted by the American Medical Association (AMA) which feared that direct federal support for medical education would place the government in the powerful position to dictate future health policy. The AMA did acquiesce, however, to the indirect federal funding of medical education through the inclusion of institutional costs in its grants for biomedical research. The suspicion of market economists that the AMA was committed to a restriction of the supply is probably an oversimplification, although the memory of the depressed 1930s when many physicians had difficulty earning a living undoubtedly influenced the leadership.

The flow of funds via the National Institutes of Health into the academic health centers intensified the pressures in favor of specialization which transformed medical education from a five-year program to one of eight or nine years of training. In the process a powerful new constituency came into being—a much strengthened Association of American Medical Colleges and its key academic supporters that operated in close league with Senator Hill and Representative Fogarty, the controllers of the federal purse for medical research.

Despite the ever larger flows of funds into the health care arena, the vast superstructure of graduate medical education—residency training—had no independent financial base. It was supported through reimbursement to teaching hospitals for patient care. I have referred to this anomalous situation as "the soft underbelly of U.S. medical education."[2]

The postwar period also witnessed a major shift in the training of nurses, from independent diploma schools of nursing based in nonprofit and government hospitals to colleges and universities where associate degree programs experienced the most rapid growth, and baccalaureate programs gained as well. Today these programs account for about four out of every five new graduates. State and federal funding also became available to educational and training programs both new and old, many located at academic health centers, for a host of allied health professionals and technicians.

Finally, in 1963, the AMA, having decided to concentrate its legislative efforts on the defeat of Medicare, acceded to direct federal support for expanding the supply of physicians and other health practitioners. The next eight years witnessed an outpouring of federal funds for new construction, support for schools in financial distress, incentives to existing schools to expand enrollments, special assistance to minorities and students from low-income families, support for residency training in family practice—all aimed at resolving the putative shortage of physicians variously estimated at between 50,000 and 80,000 and, more recently, at improving the distribution of the available supply by specialty and location.[3]

It would be hard to find even a trace of market forces operating in those halycon days when the federal government, with support from the states, poured ever larger sums into medical research and medical education to speed the discovery of new knowledge and to assure its widespread application.

We come now to the third prong—the changing contours of the demand for health care. In my view, the story begins with World War II when fifteen million men in uniform (and many of their dependents) were exposed to a high level of medical care, many for the first time in their lives. I recall being told by a much decorated sergeant who had been rotated back to the United States that his current assignment at Fort Meade, Maryland, was to instruct recruits from the Tennessee mountains in the use of soap and running water. More to the point: the U.S. army lost only 4 percent of all casualties who were reached by a medic during the course of the battle, a record that made a deep impression on the soldiers and their families.

It is often overlooked that hospital insurance did not really take off until World War II when the Wage Stabilization Board ruled that the provision of hospital benefits under new contract settlements did not violate the national wage stabilization statute. Moreover, the government provided further impetus to the growth of hospital insurance when the IRS issued a definitive ruling in 1954 that such benefits qualified as legitimate business expenses for employers and did not constitute reportable income for employees. For some three decades it has been the explicit and implicit policy of the federal government to encourage employers to improve the health benefits of their employees. It is only in the last few years that some moralistic economists have begun to rail against this "give-away," convinced that if tax deductions were capped a large part of the cost inflation in health care would vanish, an assertion that has failed to elicit any broad support among employers, trade unions, insurance companies, or other informed parties.

The striking advances in therapeutics during the postwar period were a major spur to the efforts that were mounted in the 1950s and the 1960s (Kerr-Mills, Medicare, and Medicaid) to assure that the elderly and poor would have access to acute hospitals and the same range of services enjoyed by employed workers (and their dependents). Once again, federal and state governments were in the lead to broaden and deepen the demand for health care.

The revisionist views sketched above underscore the fact that prior to World War II the health care system was in large measure a shared function of the voluntary sector, which had primary responsibility for the establishment and operation of the nation's hospitals, and of state government, which in tandem with the voluntary sector was responsible for the education and training of physicians, nurses, and other health personnel. In addition, state and local governments, again alongside the voluntary sector, provided most of the care for the poor as well as the patients suffering from serious chronic diseases such as tuberculosis and mental illness.[4]

In the postwar period it was the federal government that assumed the leadership role by encouraging the expansion of hospital insurance, contributing to hospital construction, financing biomedical research, and, after 1963, allocating large sums for medical education to expand the supply of physicians and for vast entitlement programs to provide access to care for the elderly and the poor. There are those who, like David Stockman, write about the necessity of reestablishing the market as the dominant instrumentality for the production and distribution of health care to the American people. But history does not support their argument.[5]

Let us examine the assumptions and analyses first of the market advocates, then of the proponents of a larger role for government. Clearly I must be selective in the analysts whose work is reviewed. I have deliberately skewed my selection in favor of economists with linkages to the University of Chicago which has been in the forefront of those who support the market.

A good place to begin is Milton Friedman's dissertation *Income from Independent Professional Practice,* which demonstrated, by means of a complex analytic exercise, that organized medicine, through the control of admissions to medical school, extracts rent for physicians; this is proved by the fact that physicians earn more than dentists after account is taken of differences in their period of training. Two questions: Does it make sense for a society to provide medical education for all who want to enter the profession? I doubt it. And second, will the public not be willing to pay more for an hour of work by a surgeon whose judgment and skill can make the difference between life and death, than a dentist who relieves them of a painful molar? Adam Smith had addressed this issue and had come out on the other side. No proof that he was right, but cause for caution.[6]

In the late 1950s, Reuben Kessel published his far-ranging analysis of physician behavior, indicating how organized medicine at national, state, and county levels pursued policies that reinforced the professionals' ability to act as price discriminators with the aim of blocking the introduction of new systems of health care delivery that could jeopardize fee-for-service practice.[7] Several points: the world that Kessel described with knowledge and insight is no longer the medical environment of the early 1980s. Yet fee-for-service still dominates. The monetarization of the health care system subsequent to the passage of Medicare and Medicaid put an end to the considerable amount of "unrequited" labor that physicians used to perform both in their offices and in hospitals at which they had admitting privileges. It has never been clear to me that such monetarization was an unequivocal social gain and the fact that many physicians are once again providing services free of charge, at reduced fees, or on credit for large numbers of persons who have lost their insurance coverage bears on this point.

Martin Feldstein, who also has a spiritual affinity for Chicago, has argued for years that first dollar coverage is bad and that only high copayments can control runaway hospital costs.[8] I have never understood how a market economist can deny consumers the right to buy products that they desire nor have I understood how he can reconcile high copayments with the principal of hospital insurance which was introduced for the explicit purpose of protecting the individual from sudden, large outlays.

Clark Havighurst, Chicago once removed, formulated the most cogent argument that more competition offers a superior alternative to more regulation. Until now, the arguments for and against competition in health care have been exchanged in scholarly journals to which I have of late been a prolific contributor.[9] But we will soon see the debate move from paper to reality. If I were a betting man, I would predict that increased competition will result in the flow of more resources into the health care system, a further stimulation of demand, and substantial increase in the proportion of the GNP directed to health care.

It would be wrong for me to omit Enthoven from the list of market advocates even though I know no way to tie him directly to Chicago. Three quick points: Enthoven, to his credit, believes that government must regulate competition among insurers and prepayment groups. Furthermore, he recognizes the need for special provisions (through government) to assure that persons of limited or no income have access to the system. However, much of his competitive strategy was based on the apparent success of the Federal Employee's Health Program Benefits just a short time before it revealed serious deficiencies resulting from adverse selection.[10]

A few more germane comments about the advocates of the market. They deal with health care as if it were a standardized product, with little or no consideration of the inevitable control that the physician exercises over its production and the importance that attaches to quality.[11] They also neglect or minimize the role of caring in the relation between the physician and his patient. They have no ready explanation for the slow growth of prepayment plans even after the active opposition of organized medicine had been eliminated. With the conspicuous exception of Enthoven, they are silent about how the market will provide access to essential services for the poor and the medically indigent.

The principal contribution of the market proponents to the ongoing debate about health policy has been to sharpen the analysis of the issues. In my view, however, they have contributed very little to policy guidance.

Let us now turn our attention to the exponents of social reform—among whom Michael Davis was a long-time leader—who prefer an enlarged role for government in the direction of the health care system. They have emphasized the following arenas of reform:

- The expansion of prepayment plans
- A shift in orientation from therapeutic to preventive services
- The greater use of paramedical personnel
- An enlarged role for consumers in health planning
- The introduction of national health insurance

A few brief, critical comments on each of the foregoing objectives. I have long been impressed with the indifferent performance of HMOs in Washington, D.C., and in New York City, and their relatively slow growth in their home state of California where the soil is favorable to the culture of exotic plants. I have also been impressed with the degree of continuing uncertainty about their lower hospitalization rates—a range of 10 to 40 percent is too large for comfort. Finally, cost escalation in HMOs has apparently paced cost escalation in the rest of the system.

No one will quarrel with the desirability of greater emphasis on preventive services but the question that requires answering is, just what preventive measures that have proved themselves are not being utilized more or less to the full? If the answers relate to the control of smoking, drinking, exercise, diet, then one has shifted the focus from prevention to prudence—a rarified level of behavior since the beginning of time and one which, the efforts of religious leaders and philosophers notwithstanding, we have never learned to inculcate or practice.

As a long time student of human resources, I clearly favor the optimal use of paramedical personnel. However, we now staff our health care system with fifteen ancillary workers to every one physician, up from three to one at the turn of this century. Admittedly, we could move to extend still further use of paramedics, but it is worth mentioning that Kaiser-Permanente and other large delivery systems (the military and the Veterans) have encountered difficulty in absorbing large numbers of nurse practitioners effectively.

Our recent experience with area health planning in which consumers played a prominent role must surely raise questions as to the utility of widening the scope for community participation in policy formulation. For better or worse, policy is carried out by the providers and they must be key participants in decisions to effect any significant, even minor, changes in the system. Consumers should have the right to propose changes, but only providers can implement them.

As for national health insurance (NHI), after having been on the nation's agenda since the Bull Moose campaign of 1912, it may yet stage a comeback if we fail to find viable solutions to the financing and delivery problems that appear to be multiplying. But the odds are that even under such a pessimistic scenario, we will try other nostrums before resorting to NHI.[12]

In short, I am not persuaded by the preferred solutions of the pro-government exponents. They too, like their market cousins, have little to offer by way of policy guidance.

PREMISES AND POLICY DIRECTIONS

Now that I have offered my reconstruction of the postwar evolution of the medical care system and have reviewed critically the assumptions and conclusions of the market analysts and the social reformers, it is incumbent on me to clarify my preconceptions and to set forth my recommendations for change.

To begin with my premises:

- The American people have exaggerated expectations of the potential of modern medicine, and this creates the backdrop for policies that, even if well designed and implemented, will be found wanting. The most striking and aberrant of all the conventional beliefs is that the physician has the skill and power to postpone indefinitely the patient's death. In fact, death has no part in the public's expectational system with respect to medicine.

- For a variety of reasons, some planned and other fortuitous, expenditures for the institutional sector of the health care system—hospitals and nursing homes—rose from under one-third to over one-half of total outlays in the postwar period, thereby contributing substantially to the rapid increase in costs.

- In response to the growing gap during the early postwar years between the greatly increased demand for medical care and the inelasticity in the supply of physicians, the state and federal governments undertook in the late 1950s and early 1960s a program of accelerated expansion that vastly overcompensated for any actual or presumed shortages. Even at this late date there is no general perception by the public that the country is producing too many physicians and that there are dangers, both therapeutic and economic, linked to an oversupply of physicians.

- The monetarization of the health care system that reached its apotheosis with the passage of Medicare and Medicaid obscured an earlier rule, appreciated by providers and consumers alike, that is, that all decisions about medical care must be related to economic resources. No societal function, not even medical care, education, or defense, can expect to have an unlimited credit line to the U.S. Treasury.

- The contrast between the many words that have been directed this past decade to "cost containment" and the slow progress, if any, that we have achieved should be a warning that effective responses are difficult to design and still more difficult to implement. Most of what parades as cost containment is nothing more than expenditure control.[13]

Let me identify, primarily for illustrative purposes, a few of the policy directions that flow from the foregoing premises. With respect to unbounded expenditures, the time is long overdue for the initiation of a broad discussion by the public, physicians, jurists, religious leaders, and politicians about the choices that must be permissible in the case of terminal patients. I recall a senior surgeon who revealed to me that, seeing General MacArthur in the ICU, he was unable to tell whether the General was alive or dead. The practice of hooking patients to life-prolonging but not life-improving apparatus for days, weeks, and months clearly requires reexamination, the more so because such action in many instances is not in conformity with the desires of the patient or his responsible relatives.[14]

It is over four years since GMENAC alerted the country to the substantial oversupply of physicians that looms ahead, but thus far there has been relatively little response from the medical or political leadership. Most recently, Dr. Alvin Tarlov, the chairman of GMENAC, provided an update on the problem and the steps that should be taken. But it remains to be seen whether those with the primary responsibility to act will continue to play possum.[15] Dr. Francis Moore of Harvard has made use of a spatial model to indicate the geographic location of surgical specialists through the final decades of this century, an exercise that points to the probability that as the year 2000 approaches only the smallest communities, those of 5,000 to 15,000 population, will be able to absorb any new practitioners.[16]

Multiple opportunities exist to reverse long-term trends that have favored inpatient over ambulatory care settings as the preferred locus for treatment. To begin with, variations of 100 percent or more in hospital days per 1,000 population speak to the influence of physician practice modes in determining patterns of hospital care. The frail elderly have repeatedly stressed their preferences to avoid placement in nursing homes in favor of remaining in their own homes and in their own communities. Congress recently offered terminal patients the choice of hospice care over treatment in an acute hospital. Insurance companies are belatedly writing policies with mounting incentives favoring patients who opt for the performance of specified procedures in an ambulatory setting. Massachusetts General Hospital has increased the proportion of ambulatory surgery it performs to over 30 percent of all cases. The area where we have made the least progress and where gains will come slowly is in the regionalization of highly specialized care, where duplication of costly, underutilized services is economically wasteful and carries no inconsiderable therapeutic risk.

The principal players for medical care—federal and state governments, and business and labor (through their participation in group insurance coverage)—are belatedly bestirring themselves to slow the flow of funds into health care. Walter McNerney, the Michael Davis lecturer in 1982, reviewed developments with respect to business Health Care Coalitions.[17] Since that time the Secretary of HHS has complied with the congressional directive to propose a system of prospective payment for Medicare patients, and DRGs became operational at the end of 1983. But it would be naive to expect even a much enlarged and strengthened number of business Health Care Coalitions and well-functioning DRGs to bring financial stability to the U.S. medical system. The prospective deficit for the Medicare Trust Fund for 1995 is in the $300 billion range and, as Paul Ginsburg of the Congressional Budget Office recently noted, nobody in Washington is yet facing up to this issue.[18] Congress will delay as long as possible cutting back on entitlements, levying new taxes and surcharges, raising copayments, and otherwise forcing the private sector via insurance and out-of-pocket payments to cover more of the total health care bill. But if government is to moderate its outlays, it has only two alternatives: to reduce services or to extract more funds from the nongovernmental sector—or to do both. In the event, however, that services are cut back, there is a serious danger that the poor and the medically indigent will fall through the net, an outcome to which only the most myopic would be indifferent.

Given an imbalance of dollars and services and the projection of an even greater imbalance in the years ahead, there is no easy way to restore equilibrium. No interest—the federal government, private insurance, the medical profession, the hospital establishment, the academic health centers, industry, or the trade unions—has the power to shore up the system, and surely not if each acts independently. Neither greater reliance on the market nor greater governmental direction holds the answer. Ours has long been a "mixed" health care system—supported by government, insurance, and out-of-pocket payments by consumers—with physicians and hospitals making many of the critical decisions. Academicians and policy analysts have been able to design on paper improved health care systems that are at once efficient and equitable, but they have glossed over the complexities of transforming ideas into institutions and behavior. We have no option but to continue along the path that we have been going, seeking to introduce feasible changes while preserving the many virtues of the mixed system that has evolved.

The following are some guidelines for selecting among the various changes that have been and will be proposed:

- The desirability of shifting the locus of treatment from high-cost inpatient settings to ambulatory settings
- The need for experimentation with new forms of health care delivery that advance beyond the classic two—fee-for-service and prepayment
- The urgency of measures to reduce the excess capacity of hospital beds, the proliferation of costly services, and the training of health professionals and technicians beyond present and prospective requirements of the system
- The need to assure sufficient new funds, even in a period of constricted finances, to encourage the development of the new knowledge and innovative techniques which hold the greatest promise of true long-term cost constraint
- The moral and political imperative to maintain access to the system for those who lack the means to pay their own way

It would be desirable to flesh out each of the foregoing and to indicate how the extant system might be modified so that it will move in the desired direction. In Chapter 4 I address this challenge.

In closing I will share an excerpt from the preface to *The Social Control of Business,* written by J.M. Clark some sixty years ago, in the mid-1920s, when he was a member of the Chicago Department of Economics:

The principal of free exchange offers expression to certain needs, and opportunity to certain interests to organize themselves into a sort of partial community. But this partial community of free exchange never includes all the interests that make up a complete community; and a complete community, capable of sustaining life, can never be made up of the transactions of free exchange alone. The community of free exchange cannot maintain itself except in the enveloping medium of a broader community life, which furnishes the conditions on which free exchange depends and stands ready to do the innumerable things it leaves undone and to care for the interests which it neglects. [19]

2

Monetarization of Medical Care

Close observers of the health care system, among them Arnold Relman and David Rogers,[1] are alarmed at how fast American medicine appears to be turning from a profession into a business. The evidence of history and economics suggests that a related and more pervasive trend, the monetarization of medical care, has been proceeding apace for the past several decades and dominates the present scene.

Monetarization can be defined as the rapid penetration since 1950 of the "money economy" into all facets of the health care system. Its influence is reflected in the following developments: the order of magnitude of growth in the financial dimensions of academic health centers; the shift from voluntary to employed physicians in large teaching hospitals; the payment of reasonable stipends to house staff; the marked decline in the role of philanthropy in meeting the operating deficits and the capital needs of nonprofit hospitals; and the substantial reduction in unrequited services by physicians, especially after the introduction of Medicare and Medicaid. This process of monetarization has set the stage for the explosive growth of for-profit medicine.

A glimpse into history reveals large-scale changes in the traditional system that are essential to understanding both the present predicament and the outlook for the future. In 1940 philanthropy accounted for 24 percent of the total operating budget of nonprofit hospitals in New York City; by 1948 it had dropped to 17 percent.[2] According to the United Hospital Fund of New York, its share is now barely 1 percent. The last figure underestimates the amount of free care that hospitals and physicians continue to provide to the sick poor through cross-subsidization and unre-

Originally published in *New England Journal of Medicine* 310:8 (1162–65), May 3, 1984. Reprinted by permission.

quited services, but the volume is greatly reduced from that of decades past.

Before World War II, physicians in training—interns and residents—were required to live in the hospital and were on duty every other night. Some received a small cash stipend, but many worked for room, board, and laundry. Interns were not permitted to marry, and fellows did not earn enough to marry. Physicians who sought admitting privileges at a prestigious hospital had to work in its clinics for a period of years, donating several half-days per week; if appointed to the staff, they continued to donate several half-days per week to care for patients on the wards. Most physicians adjusted their office fees for those unable to meet them in full.

One more critical fact: capital funds for new construction, expansion, and modernization were raised by the trustees of voluntary hospitals from among themselves, their friends, legacies from the wealthy, and on special occasions, from a broad community fund-raising effort.

Up to the beginning of World War II, American medicine was partly monetarized, partly eleemosynary. Thereafter, a major expansion in hospital insurance and the long upward trend in real family income set the stage for the complete monetarization of health care, the final phase of which followed the enactment of the Medicare and Medicaid programs in 1965.

The monetarization process was speeded by the changing relationships in supply and demand between those who sought medical care and those who provided it. Patients with more income and better insurance coverage found it easier to seek and pay for medical care. Hospitals treated fewer nonpaying patients, largely as a result of the rapid spread of insurance. With more revenue and fewer bad debts, hospitals were able to pay nurses and nonprofessional personnel higher, if not yet competitive, wages and salaries. The charitable element in hospital operations dwindled as hospitals became more fully integrated into the money economy.

Several additional points: government financing became available for the first time (through the Hill-Burton Act, 1946) to assist voluntary hospitals, primarily in small communities, to meet their capital needs; substantial funding from the National Institutes of Health enabled many academic health centers to become major educational, research, and service enterprises with budgets ten or twenty times larger than those of the prewar era; Blue Cross, commercial insurance, and selected government financing programs were willing and able to cover the rapidly expanding costs of graduate medical education through patient reimbursement.

Even more striking was the decline of philanthropy as the principal source of capital funding. Third-party payers accepted funded depreciation as a reimbursable charge. When voluntary hospitals needed additional sums for expansion or modernization, they went to the capital markets to borrow, using their anticipated future reimbursements as guarantee of their credit-worthiness.

As general practitioners and specialists found it increasingly easy to earn good livelihoods, they curtailed their hours of work and particularly the amount of time that they donated to hospitals for the care of the poor. Residents provided more and more of the free and below-cost services that voluntary hospitals continued to render, particularly in their expanding emergency rooms.

The passage of the Medicare and Medicaid legislation in 1965 transformed the great majority of the poor into paying patients, thereby vastly increasing the flow of funds into the health care system. Hospitals, physicians, and the rapidly increasing number of nursing homes were the principal beneficiaries. Together, they accounted by the mid-1970s for close to 70 percent of all health care expenditures.[3]

Cost-based or charge-based reimbursement encouraged hospitals to increase and upgrade the services they offered, with almost complete protection against financial loss. In this unconstrained financial environment, for-profit medical enterprises, particularly in the South and West, found many opportunities to start and expand highly profitable operations.

Another facet of the monetarization process dates from the early postwar years, when first the Veterans Administration and later the large municipal hospitals that delivered acute care to the indigent contracted with the nation's medical schools for affiliations.[4] These affiliations provided medical schools with more sites for graduate training and faculty positions and made additional funding available for research.

Three other developments should be noted. First of all, the many new and enlarged sources of funding were the primary cause for the steep inflation in health care prices that outpaced the gains in the Consumer Price Index throughout most of the past three decades. In 1950, expenditures for health care in the United States totaled $13 billion, or 4.5 percent of the Gross National Product. The latest figure available (1982) is $322 billion, or 10.5 percent of a much larger base.[5]

Second, the combination of an elongated period of graduate training before entry into independent practice, together with an improved outlook for professional earnings, raised the expectations of the postwar generation of physicians about their future incomes. By the mid-1970s, specialists in training—particularly those in the procedure-oriented specialties—could reasonably anticipate earning at least $100,000 within a few years of board certification.

The third salient development can be classified as the practice of defensive medicine and the associated phenomenon of steeply rising professional-liability costs. The malpractice insurance premium for a neurosurgeon in New York City is in the $70,000 range at present. That means that a young neurosurgeon starting out in independent practice faces a prospective outlay of $150,000 per year in terms of office rent, liability coverage, and other expenses—before seeing the first patient.

The thrust of the foregoing is to underscore that the financial dimensions of medical practice underwent a major transformation in the postwar era as a consequence of the many changes in the provision, distribution, and payment of services. The proportion of contributions by philanthropy to hospital operating and capital requirements has been greatly reduced, and the same is true of the voluntary services of physicians, inside and outside of hospitals. The nursing care given by nuns in Catholic hospitals (an important form of unrequited service in earlier decades) has all but disappeared.

The scale of this transformation was suggested at a recent symposium at the Columbia-Presbyterian Medical Center (New York City) by Dr. Henry Aranow, who noted that in the late 1930s, when he joined the staff of Presbyterian Hospital, a patient with advanced pulmonary disease who was admitted for pneumonia would die within a day or two, having run up a terminal hospital bill of $8 to $12. Today, this bill could, under special circumstances, reach $100,000. Overall there has been an approximately fivefold increase in real per capita outlays for health care in the past third of a century. It is this fact that has forced the issue of management to the fore.

To be concrete: a major academic health center with its principal teaching hospital has annual outlays in the $200 million range, the hospital usually accounting for between one-half and two-thirds of the total. A very large medical complex, such as the Mayo Clinic, with its large teaching and substantial research component, has annual outlays in excess of $400 million (excluding the independent activities of its affiliates, St. Mary's and Methodist Hospitals). Whatever their designation—public, private, nonprofit, voluntary, or for-profit—medical complexes with annual expenditures in excess of $100 million, as well as those operating on a more modest scale, need strong management to perform their multiple functions of education, research, and service efficiently, and at the same time to make effective use of the resources at their command.

It should no longer come as a surprise that for-profit medical enterprises have been able to make rapid headway during the past decade and a half—buying up existing hospitals; raising capital on the equity markets to build new hospitals in preferred locations where there is little risk of bad debt; and managing hospitals in middle-income and upper-income areas where patients, most of them heavily insured, will not object to paying a little more for comfort and service, even if they get no more and often a little less in the quality of professional care. Hospital chains have been in a particularly strong position to develop space, equipment, personnel standards, and purchasing arrangements, each of which may give them a slight edge over the single, freestanding, nonprofit hospital.

Certain ineluctable forces have drawn medical care ever more deeply into the vortex of the money economy, where management techniques must aim at the preservation and enhancement of capital. If we look ahead, these forces appear even more powerful. Consider the following: the high cost of introducing and perfecting new technology; the opportunities for corporate enterprises to attract and retain both young and mature physicians who will be available, even eager, for salaried employment; the current unbundling of services, which is likely to accelerate as entrepreneurial physicians see opportunities to improve their earnings by undertaking more diagnostic work and other procedures in their offices, in preference to the hospital; the introduction of DRGs (reimbursement based on diagnosis-related groups), which will inevitably lead to tighter hospital controls over modes of physician practice, mediated by ever more elaborate computerization; and the recent emphasis by both for-profit and nonprofit hospitals on marketing policies and diversification, which are leading to links with other health care providers, particularly physician groups, nursing homes, and hospices, and intensifying the need for skilled management if the hospitals are to survive and prosper.

Although I have singled out the impact of monetarization on the hospital sector, it must be noted that physicians in and outside of hospitals are the critical providers of care. Relman is surely right in being deeply concerned about the growing conflict between medical ethics and money-making goals,[6] an issue that the American Medical Association—and I would add, state licensing officials and other regulatory bodies, both public and private—should keep under close surveillance. To view the practice of medicine as just another business undertaking like retailing or banking is to be blind to the role of agency in the work of a professional. To rely on the market to discipline money-grubbing professionals is to overestimate what the market should be asked to do or is capable of doing.[7]

There are further indications of the increasing importance of the money economy in the delivery of health care services. The continuing growth of for-profit chains has already had the inevitable consequence of stimulating freestanding nonprofit hospitals to explore alternative means of affiliation and merger so that they will be better able to stave off their increasingly strong competitors.[8] In this connection, it is worth recalling the point made in an address to the Association of American Medical Colleges several years ago by Dr. Robert Heyssel, the president of Johns Hopkins Hospital, that little difference remains between a for-profit hospital raising money on the equity markets and a nonprofit hospital forced to meet the interest payments on its bond issue.[9] Each is subservient to the lender.

The involvement of the nation's medical supply companies in a proposal for the development of a commission, drawn from the for-profit and nonprofit sectors and government, to explore alternative ways of rationalizing the introduction of new costly technology bespeaks their concern that innovation may become the victim of cost containment not that the uncontrolled market with a limitless stream of new funds is a thing of the past.[10]

Finally, the tightening of the capital markets for institutional financing will force hospital leaders to pay more attention to financial controls and improved market strategies aimed at assuring the survival and vitality of the community hospitals and medical centers that are the backbone of sophisticated medical care for the American people. The cumulative effect of these potent forces has been at the heart of the continued monetarization of American medicine.

Two overlapping issues must be sharply differentiated: the broad consequences of the almost total monetarization of our health care system, and the role of for-profit enterprises in shaping its future. There is no possible way for any large provider to escape the dictates of the dollar. Congress has begun to explore alternatives to the large deficit in the Medicare Trust Fund that looms ahead; business coalitions are intensifying their efforts to moderate increases in their health insurance premiums; state governments, such as those of California and Massachusetts, have resorted to radical innovations to rein in their steeply rising outlays for health services. Nonprofit hospitals are merging or are joining chains (or both) and are intensifying their marketing efforts to assure themselves of a steady flow of patients. In the meantime, for-profit enterprises continue to expand through the purchase or construction of additional hospitals and ambulatory facilities and through a wide array of other approaches, from the establishment of new health maintenance organizations to working out ingenious arrangements with physicians to lease back equipment.

The policy arena is beginning to change. Congress acted recently to limit the returns on capital that would be approved by Medicare for reimbursement of for-profit hospitals, and warned that such returns might be completely disallowed after 1986. Several states, including New York, Massachusetts, Maryland, and New Jersey, have introduced a method of hospital reimbursement in which a portion of the total reimbursement pool is sequestered for distribution among the participating hospitals in proportion to the bad debts that they have incurred in treating the indigent.

The recently initiated DRG system will act to constrain for-profit hospitals from heavy reliance on ancillary charges as a source of revenue. A considerable number of municipalities and counties that are transferring their facilities to a for-profit chain have stipulated in their contracts of sale that the purchaser must provide a designated amount of free or subsidized care to the locality's indigent citizens.

Raising new money in the bond market is currently more difficult than it has been, and if a number of hospitals start to default, as may happen in the years ahead, all institutions, including the for-profit chains, will encounter difficulties when they attempt to obtain additional funding for continued expansion. Moreover, they will have to compete with some strong nonprofit chains that may be equally attractive to bondholders.

We have had relatively little success during the past decade in moderating advances in hospital costs, but even if the first-generation DRG system fails to accomplish what its proponents envisage, by the third generation we should have a better functioning system in place. The tighter the system is controlled, the less scope there will be for for-profit institutions to exploit hitherto advantageous niches.

Until now, the argument between critics and defenders of the growth of the for-profit sector in medical care has been formulated in terms of the sources of its profits. Relman maintains, with considerable merit, that these profits reflect entrepreneurial practices—the buying and selling of assets, "creaming" of the market, and avoiding unprofitable activities such as teaching and care for the poor.[11] The defenders emphasize gains from access to capital, improved planning and operating systems, and more professional management.[12] From the perspective of this review of the monetarization of the U.S. health care system, the answer is to be found in the opportunities created by faulty public policy, primarily through reimbursement, for those with money-making proclivities to establish a strong niche in what was formerly a quasi-eleemosynary sector. The American public cannot continue indefinitely down the path that it has been following—that is, to devote an ever larger share of its Gross National Product to health care. But only the naive believe that the goals that must be pursued—innovation, quality, access, and equity at an affordable cost—can be achieved either by greater reliance on the for-profit sector or by radically constraining its growth.

To secure its long-term financial foundation, American medicine will require a combination of political leadership and professional cooperation that is not yet visible on the horizon. The great danger is that such cooperation will be delayed past the point at which intervention can be effective.

3

Cost Containment: Imaginary and Real

Public opinion surveys during the past decade have placed cost containment at the head of the nation's health agenda.[1] The concept of cost containment as it is currently used implies expenditure reductions, efficiency gains in the use of resources, or a restructuring of health care delivery in which fewer interventions result in no diminution in health status. Health policy analysts of different persuasions seek support for the reforms they propose on the grounds that they will contribute to cost containment.[2]

THE MANY MEANINGS OF COST CONTAINMENT

For heuristic purposes, I will distinguish five major areas in which the concept of cost containment has wide currency: government expenditure policies, government regulatory policies, health insurance and other prepayment mechanisms, health care delivery systems, and medical practice. There is an element of arbitrariness in the choice of rubrics under which the following issues are discussed, but their assignment has no analytic importance.

Government Expenditure Policies

When congressmen vote to reduce federal expenditures for Medicare and Medicaid through a series of devices, such as restricting the number of people on the Medicaid rolls, increasing the deductibles and copayments that Medicare beneficiaries must cover, or narrowing the services for which Medicare will reimburse, they believe they are contributing to cost containment. These actions do reduce the short-term costs of medical care

Originally published in *New England Journal of Medicine* 308:20 (1220–24), May 19, 1983. Reprinted by permission.

covered by the federal government. Some of these costs will be shifted to other payers; but if not, what are the likely effects of such a reduction on the total output of health care services, and what are the long-term consequences for the health of the affected groups?

We can assume that people who are no longer eligible for Medicaid will still be treated if they have a heart attack, are hit by a truck, or have hepatitis. Physicians and hospitals will treat these persons even though federal and state governments no longer cover all or part of their bills. Total health care costs have not been contained; they have simply been shifted from the federal and state governments to the private sector—to the medically indigent, to physicians, to hospitals, and to philanthropy.

It is doubtful, however, that the private sector will be able or willing to cover the deep cuts in government outlays that now loom on the horizon, especially tax dollars that heretofore were spent on care for the poor and the elderly. Therefore, some of those who were previously entitled to subsidized health services will no longer have access to them or will be able to receive only fewer services or services of lesser quality. This raises the question of whether reduced access to health care for increasing numbers of the poor and the medically indigent may result in greater costs over the long term.[3]

A related example: Many state legislatures have recently reduced the number of persons on their Medicaid rolls who are eligible for care in nursing homes. This has reduced the rate of current and prospective state spending for health care, which many interpret as cost containment. But if a working member of the family must resign his or her job to stay home and care for the patient, the total social costs of reducing admissions to nursing homes may not be reduced or may actually show an increase.

Government Regulatory Policies

In the late 1970s President Carter twice sought congressional approval for an annual ceiling on the degree of increase in reimbursement rates for Medicare and Medicaid and on total national capital expenditures for health facilities,[4] on the assumption that total outlays for national health care would decelerate and lead to cost containment. Even if the President's expectations had been realized, the claim of cost containment would not necessarily have been justified. These regulations might have forced hospitals to delay admissions, use antiquated equipment, or turn away patients who could not pay. Therefore, it would be a misuse of language to talk of such actions as cost containment.

In response to a congressional directive motivated by the need for cost containment, the Department of Health and Human Services recently introduced a system of prospective payment based on diagnosis-related groups (DRGs) for hospitals that treat Medicare patients.[5] It is too early to know whether the DRG system will provide a sound basis for a national system of prospective budgeting; whether such a system will in fact create incentives for efficiency; whether it will prove equitable both to institutions that have been well managed and to those that have been poorly managed; and what the administrative costs required to operate it will be. Not until we have answers to these and other questions that will surface only after the system becomes fully operational will we know whether prospective budgeting based on DRGs is indeed a cost containment mechanism.[6]

Another instance of government regulation in pursuit of cost containment has been the requirement that hospitals obtain a certificate of need to purchase and use a CT scanner—an effort aided and abetted by leaders of medicine who fear the use, overuse, and misuse of this new technology with its high operating costs. Many large hospitals were denied a certificate of need and were told to use a CT machine at a neighboring institution. Often, however, these decisions did not give adequate consideration to the accessibility of the scanner, the additional costs to the referring hospital generated by scheduling delays, and the dangers of transporting seriously ill patients. Worst of all, the denial of a certificate of need on the basis of cost containment ignored potential long-term benefits of the new technology, such as the substantial gains from limiting invasive imaging, the likelihood of rapid improvements in technique that would follow its adoption, and price declines that would follow its widespread sale.[7]

Health Insurance and Other Prepayment Mechanisms

An early concern with cost containment led Martin Feldstein, currently chairman of the Council of Economic Advisers, to advocate that the nation's reliance on prepayment for hospital care be modified so that patients would be required to pay a large sum for their hospitalization, as a means of discouraging their use of unnecessary or expensive accommodations and procedures.[8] Realizing that the physician, not the consumer, usually determines the range and depth of the hospital services that the patient receives, Alain Enthoven later recommended, in the name of cost containment, imposition of a ceiling on the federal government's subsidy for health insurance,[9] as the preferred method for encouraging the economic use of health care.

A recent study by the Rand Corporation of the effect of prepayment coverage on use of health care facilities provides support to advocates of cost containment who favor deductibles and copayments at the point of use of medical or hospital care.[10] But as Rashi Fein made clear in an editorial in the *New England Journal of Medicine* that accompanied the release of the Rand findings, judgments about cost containment must be held in abeyance until we know whether patients who use fewer health services because of larger copayments have poorer health.[11]

At the time Medicare was placed on the statute books, the political leadership stated that the appropriation would cover most of the health care expenditures of the elderly. Currently, it covers only 44 percent of their annual expenditures,[12] and this fraction will surely decline in the future. At what point will the promise of Medicare have evaporated in the pursuit of cost containment?

A reading of the recommendations advanced by many advocates of stringent cost containment leaves the impression that they are unwilling to face up to a basic dilemma: Prepayment may well encourage a higher level of demand for health care, but all advanced nations have determined that prepayment (or entitlement for the entire population) is the only effective way to protect the public against the high costs of hospitalization.[13]

Health Care Delivery Systems

Advocates of prepaid health care delivery contend that health maintenance organizations are a preferred way to deliver services because they contain costs through reduced hospital admissions and through emphasis on preventive services. The evidence on the expanded use and effectiveness of preventive services is more problematic than savings from reduced hospitalization.[14] Some reports indicate that the savings from prepayment over fee-for-service are in the 10 to 15 percent range; others estimate that these savings are in the 30 to 40 percent range. If the savings are in the lower range, many persons would prefer to see their private physicians by appointment rather than to spend hours awaiting their turn to be treated by different physicians on successive visits to a clinic.

During the past decade the growth of health maintenance organizations has been favored as a result of lessened hostility from organized medicine, federal subsidies, and the availability of private capital for new ventures. Still, their rate of growth has been modest, and most observers now believe that health maintenance organizations will not be able to make a major contribution to cost containment by 1990.[15]

In 1974 the minister of national health and welfare in Canada, Marc Lalonde, put forward in the name of cost containment the radical proposal that the flow of public resources be shifted from curative to preventive medicine.[16] Since that time, various leaders of health policy in the United States, including the former secretary of the Department of Health and Human Services, have stressed the aspects of prevention that can contribute to cost containment. So far these proponents have not specified which therapeutic interventions would be reduced or eliminated. Moreover, the proposal gives short shrift to the major social costs involved in the constraint of personal freedom necessary to reduce or eliminate smoking, alcohol abuse, and other forms of substance abuse and to ensure that people engage in regular exercise and control their weight.

Medical Practice

Leaders of the medical profession in Europe disagree about the relative value of surgery or drugs as the treatment of choice for patients with arteriosclerotic heart disease.[17] Although the arguments continue, the frequency of high-cost surgical interventions increases. From the standpoint of cost containment, the lack of clear-cut evidence that surgery contributes in most cases to a prolongation of the patient's life would lend support to the alternative therapy based on drugs. But there are other considerations, such as whether patients who have had successful bypass surgery have less pain and fear and are better able to continue working than those who are treated with medication alone. These are critical variables that need to be included in an assessment of surgery versus drugs. Such an assessment must precede any attempt at cost containment.

The usual explanation for the disproportionately high use of hospital-based renal dialysis is the power and avarice of institutional providers.[18] That may be part of the story, but it is surely not all of it. A shift to home-based dialysis would reduce Medicare's expenditures, but before such a move could be defined as cost containment it would be necessary to answer several questions. How many patients would be able to undergo dialysis at home? Would other members of the household be able to handle the burden? Would the medical outcomes be the same? Without an assessment of the additional burdens to the patient and members of the family and an evaluation of the outcome, one would not be justified in considering the shift to home dialysis as a clear-cut base of cost containment.

"Surgicenters" provide another illustration of potential, not proved, cost containment. Superficially, it would appear that a shift from multiple days of inpatient treatment in an acute care hospital to ambulatory surgery, in which the patient goes home a few hours after surgery, is a clear-cut instance of cost containment. It may be, but we cannot be sure. It is necessary to determine whether the new surgicenter beds have led to a corresponding reduction in the community's inpatient bed capacity or whether they have been added to it. A similar inquiry would have to be made with respect to ancillary equipment and staffing. The most important principle here is that surgery in the United States, under the leadership of the American College of Surgeons, has established a high standard of quality control. In hospitals, surgeons are responsible to their peers.

Unless peer control were extended to the surgicenter, total costs, measured in both dollars and human terms, might increase. If that were to happen, it would clearly be wrong to consider the expansion of surgicenters as cost containment.

During the 1960s the nation made major efforts to expand the supply of physicians and other health personnel, with the expectation that as the number of providers increased, the costs of health care would be reduced. Economists were in the vanguard of those who insisted that expanding the supply of physicians would lead to a reduction in fees and that further economies could be achieved by enlarging the number of paraprofessionals.[19] But the expected gains in cost containment did not occur, because those who espoused the supply side approach did not distinguish between unit and total costs of physician services and because most paraprofessionals were added to the medical team without any reduction in physician personnel.[20]

The only reasonable conclusion to be drawn from the foregoing is that cost containment in health care is an elusive concept; it is difficult to define and even more difficult to apply.

TOWARD EFFECTIVE COST CONTAINMENT

Effective cost containment must take account of both sides of the equation: outputs as well as inputs, total as well as unit costs, and long-term as well as short-term results. In the light of these criteria, can we identify specific programs and policies that would qualify as effective cost containment? The answer is an unequivocal yes, and a few illustrations follow.

In passing the tax reform bill in the summer of 1982, Congress provided an option for terminally ill patients: Medicare would henceforth pay for their care in hospices or in acute care hospitals. Although exercise of the hospice option requires that the patient forego treatment in an acute care facility for a time, a shift in favor of hospice care (with corresponding reductions in acute care hospital beds) could lead to a lower total outlay for terminal care.[21]

Most regional and local differences in the average cost per hospital admission (adjusted for age and other relevant demographic and diagnostic variables) are not associated with ascertainable differences in patient outcomes or satisfaction. Therefore, a combination of incentives and pressures on physicians and hospitals that currently have fees and costs far above the norm to move in stages toward the mean would contribute to cost containment. Parenthetically, in my view, it would be easier to achieve lower costs through regulation than through competition.

On the basis of the experience of health maintenance organizations and other group practice arrangements, a shift from inpatient to ambulatory care should moderate total outlays without any diminution in patient satisfaction and health status. There are also gains in cost containment to be achieved through a strengthening of home health care services as a substitute for institutional care.

The ratio of physicians to population is likely to rise from 200 to 280 per 100,000 by the century's end. Therefore, we cannot expect a reduction in the number of physicians relative to other less extensively trained health professionals. However, if it eventually occurred, such a reduction could contribute to cost containment.[22] Improved use of personnel would have to await a reduction in the number of newly graduated physicians, as well as innovative and more effective forms of service delivery. Under favorable conditions, however, new forms of staffing and service delivery could contribute to cost containment.[23]

No innovation could make a greater contribution to cost containment over the long term than an investment by the American people in maintaining their own health through alterations in their personal behavior.[24] This change cannot be effected by legislation, as Lalonde believed; it depends on long-term changes in education, reflected in new life-styles and behavioral patterns.

Health analysts and health managers should accelerate their search for effective cost containment. But they must not assume that legislative or financial gimmickry, such as reducing the Medicaid rolls, using certificates of need to deny hospitals the right to buy new equipment, insisting on more copayments from patients at hospitalization, and placing a ceiling on reimbursements for Medicare or Medicaid, will result in effective cost containment. At best, such actions can constrain the expenditures of selected payers, particularly government. At worst, the cost savings will mask the fact that they result in a decline in services for the indigent. Reductions in expenditures that result in lowering the level and quality of health care, particularly for the poor, should not be confused with cost containment. Such confusion is a perversion of language and logic.

What then is true cost containment? It is simply this: a reduced inflow of real resources into the health care system without a diminution in useful output that would adversely affect the satisfaction of patients or their health status. The best prospects for true cost containment include professional leadership that eliminates the use of resources for procedures of dubious value and constrains new outlays until new technology has been assessed, adoption by insurers and payers of incentive systems that favor the reduction and elimination of underused and duplicative costly services, shifts from more to less costly settings (inpatient to ambulatory), and education and other approaches that encourage people to play a more active part in the protection of their health and in the judicious use of the health care system.

4

The Delivery System: What Lies Ahead?

The more complex the world becomes, the greater the pressures on leaders, academicians, and analysts to develop simplified models to communicate with the public whose support they seek. Such models can often yield important inferences, their results and recommendations can be broadly communicated from the few to the many, and the absence of comprehensive data to support their inferences and conclusions is easy to conceal. Partly because data are costly to collect and are often not disseminated, few judgments in the public policy arena are decided on "the facts" alone. Accordingly, most policy debates deteriorate into a choice among several highly simplified models.

Nowhere has the power of a model been more potent than in the case of the "free market." Despite powerful evidence to the contrary, successive presidents, from Kennedy to Reagan, have proceeded on the assumption that the United States is a free market economy. Currently, the not-for-profit sector (government and nonprofit institutions) accounts for more than one-quarter of the GNP and about one-third of all employment. And many industries are dominated by large corporations whose aim is to control rather than be controlled by the market. A critical question that is seldom raised, however, is whether the model of the competitive market fits the reality not just in some but in most sectors of the economy. And what I especially question herein is whether the health care system has ever truly functioned—or would be able to function effectively—in a free market, or competitive, framework.

MODELS VERSUS REALITY

In decades past, philanthropy played the dominant role in the construction and often also the financing of local hospitals. Although the latter is

Originally published as "The Delivery of Health Care: What Lies Ahead?" *Inquiry* 20:3 (201–17), Fall 1983. Reprinted by permission.

no longer the case, the long dominance of philanthropy should alert us to the questionable assumption made by many leaders of the procompetition approach that the competitive market earlier governed the provision of hospital care. It did not. The United States has thus far had little experience with price competition in the health care market. This is not to say that price competition has been totally absent, but its reach has been limited.

If the health care market does not conform to the model of the competitive market, what alternative construct should be applied? A pluralistic model is required that makes room for the changing roles of the following major elements: philanthropy, government, nonprofit and commercial insurers, and the consumer. If one limits the period of inspection to the post-World War II era—that is, from 1950 to 1983, a third of a century—one can trace the expansion and transformation of the U.S. health care system in terms of the altered roles of these four principal actors.

For example, in 1950 Medicare and Medicaid did not exist. The legislation establishing these programs was passed in 1965. By 1980, a decade and a half later, federal outlays for these programs alone amounted to $49.5 billion, which represented 80 percent of all federal outlays for personal health care and about one out of every four dollars of all personal health care expenditures.

If the payments by government are added to those of insurance, one finds that third-party payers accounted for 30.9 percent of all personal health expenditures in 1950 and 66.2 percent in 1980. Narrowing the focus to outlays for hospitals, the single largest component of personal health expenditures, the respective figures are 66.7 percent in 1950 and 89.7 percent in 1980. In the latter year, the consumer paid no more than 9.1 percent out-of-pocket for hospital care, philanthropy being responsible for the small residual.

The dominance of philanthropy in earlier decades and more recently of federal and local governments as sources of capital funds for hospitals and medical schools suggests the need for caution in applying the competitive model to the health care sector. In truly competitive markets, it is the entrepreneur, not government, that provides the required capital funds.

Thus, the health sector did not conform to the model of the competitive market in 1950 and it clearly does not conform to it today. Further, government has played the major role in the expansion and transformation of the health sector during the past three decades. These considerations, as well as the continually shifting relations among the three sections—private, nonprofit, and government—and the further differentiations that emerge when one distinguishes capital investments from operating activities, underscore the inappropriateness of using the competitive market model to assess the performance of the health care system.

The proponents of greater competition, nonetheless, believe that the steep rise in health care costs that has created increasing strain for providers, payers, and consumers can best be moderated by expanding the opportunities for market forces to exercise greater influence on the market behavior of all participants. Whether such a policy has merit depends on a prior analysis of the causes for the steep acceleration in costs, the adaptability of the dominant health care institutions to the changing environment, and possible alternatives to a competitive market solution.

COST CONTAINMENT CHURNINGS

The principal advocates of change in the health care sector have been legislators, primarily members of Congress, who have become increasingly restive about the uncontrollable growth in federal outlays for Medicare and Medicaid, as well as for other federally funded health care programs. In 1972, as health care costs continued to rise, Congress explored new ways to bring them under control. Specifically, it sought to slow the expansion of hospital capacity by stipulating that it would provide reimbursement for the care of Medicare and Medicaid patients in newly constructed beds only if they had been authorized by a certificate of need (CON) from the state. In the same year, Congress enacted the professional standards review organization legislation that encouraged the organization of physician groups to monitor hospital admissions and utilization. Several years of experience, however, have yielded little or no firm evidence that either of these efforts had an appreciable effect on outlays for hospital care.

In 1977, Alain Enthoven put forth his Consumer Choice Health Plan (CCHP), which looked to a reconstruction of the health care market over a period of years primarily through an expanding role for competition. CCHP can be viewed as the second stage of an effort that the federal government undertook in 1973 when it passed the initial legislation to encourage the growth of health maintenance organizations (HMOs) by making available federal grants and loans for planning and start-up expenditures. The proponents of HMOs, including Enthoven, pointed to important gains inherent in comprehensive prepaid health delivery schemes: lower costs resulting from a much reduced rate of hospitalization, engaging the self-interest of participating physicians to control costs, and the opportunity to shift the focus of care from inpatient curative treatment to outpatient preventive services. HMOs and other prepaid practice arrangements appeared to be the hope and promise of the future.

HMOs, however, have grown relatively slowly, and the best-informed analysts question whether their present level of enrollment, 4 percent to 5 percent of the population, will exceed 10 percent or 12 percent by 1990. In light of this anticipated modest growth, there is limited prospect for HMOs to exercise in the near and medium term a significant constraint on spiraling health care costs.

The Reagan administration, even in its early enthusiasm and support for the new procompetition initiatives to control health care expenditures, recognized that the potential gains would at best take a long time to achieve. Faced with an uncontrollable budget and projections of rapidly rising outlays for health care in the years ahead, the administration sought to cap its future commitments.

The Budget Reconciliation Act of 1982 (H.R. 4961) made cuts projected to reduce hospital reimbursements by a total of $6.6 billion over fiscal years 1983–1985. Overall savings for Medicare and Medicaid (hospital and other components) were projected to amount to $3.2 billion in fiscal year 1983. But the most effective actions taken thus far by the federal government involve the successive tightening of administrative regulations governing the conditions under which it reimburses providers for Medicare and Medicaid. In their absence, the expenditures of the federal government for health care would be considerably above their present high level. One must quickly add that the spiraling costs have not been brought under control; at best their rate of increase has been blunted.

In a few states, such as New York, Connecticut, and Maryland, state regulatory agencies have been given broad powers by the legislature to control hospital costs, which consume between 20 percent and 40 percent of all Medicaid expenditures, both for Medicaid eligibles and for Medicare patients who require supplementation by Medicaid. However, the states that became deeply involved in hospital cost controls had broader objectives than moderating the increase in their Medicaid liability. They were primarily concerned with moderating increases in hospital reimbursements including those authorized for Blue Cross Plans, in many areas the principal private sector payer. Although the federal efforts at cost control had proved largely unsuccessful, the most recent studies suggest that these three states, as well as several others, may have become reasonably effective in slowing the rise in their hospital costs.

Recently the federal government has issued waivers to a few states that enable them to restrict the right of Medicaid eligibles to free choice of physician and permit the states to designate the providers from whom the beneficiaries receive services. The states, including California, that are experimenting with this approach expect preferred providers to be more cost effective.

A related problem concerns hospitals that are under severe pressure to provide a large amount of free or partial-pay care to the poor and the medically indigent. Several states, such as New York, New Jersey, and Maryland, provide special funding to such institutions or have established a mechanism for allocating the costs of uncovered care among all payers, including government, insurance, and self-paying patients.

Various Blue Cross and Blue Shield Plans, commercial insurers, and selected employer and labor groups have exercised pressure on providers to slow the rise in their health care outlays. These interventions have covered a wide terrain, including the disallowance of reimbursement for days of care in excess of established standards or for procedures that professional leaders have defined as ineffective; limiting reimbursement for certain procedures to low-cost (ambulatory) settings; introducing new benefits to encourage the use of less expensive facilities such as home health care or hospices; encouraging the development of HMOs as an alternative to traditional fee-for-service care; rigorous auditing of provider claims to discourage fraud and abuse; and still other approaches including the encouragement of hospital mergers and closures.

But constraining costs and outlays is not the only challenge that the health care system confronts. It must seek also to maintain a viable hospital system, to adapt to the much larger number of physicians who will enter professional practice, and to make effective use of the new knowledge and technology that will become available to improve the quality of care. If the 1970s have taught us anything, it is that solutions come hard.

THE HUMAN RESOURCES OUTLOOK

With the demand for medical services rising rapidly as a result of substantial gains in family income reinforced by the growth of insurance, public pressures for expanding the physician supply increased during the last third of a century. The 1950s saw a response from some states and additional, if indirect, funding for medical education from the federal government's burgeoning support for biomedical research. Philanthropy also made a modest contribution. As a result, the number of physicians expanded to keep pace with the increasing population. In the early 1960s, the last barriers to direct federal support of medical education were eliminated and the new flow of federal dollars added to the growing outlays by state governments finally produced a marked enlargement in the training structure. The numbers of medical schools rose from 90 in 1960 to 126 at the beginning of the 1980s. There were corresponding increases in enrollments from 32,000 to 65,000 and in annual graduates from 7,500 to 15,700. Simultaneously with this expansion in the domestic medical education structure, the United States admitted and absorbed large numbers of graduates of foreign medical schools, with the result that between 1960 and 1980, the ratio of physicians to population increased roughly from 150 to 200 per 100,000, or by one-third. By 1990, the ratio is projected to exceed 240 per 100,000, which will represent an increase of 60 percent since the start of the expansionary trend thirty years earlier.

During the 1960s and early 1970s when it was believed that the country confronted a serious shortage of physicians, the federal government, state governments, and the private sector took steps to encourage the training of physician assistants and nurse practitioners. The rationale was that such personnel could stretch the supply of physicians by serving as initial contacts for many patients entering the health care system and by assuming responsibility, usually under supervision, for routine medical procedures.

If one postulates that the physician has been and will remain the fulcrum of the health care system, the likelihood of an emerging "surplus" of 70,000 physicians by 1990, as estimated by the Graduate Medical Education National Advisory Committee, will have a significant impact on the future of health care delivery.

A rapidly increasing supply of physicians, although resulting in lower average incomes, could also produce a substantial rise in total health care costs. One should not assume that the large increase in the physician supply will result in the overtreatment of patients, although such may turn out to be the case. A more likely outcome is that physicians will provide the public with services that they could not obtain if their supply remained taut, such as care during evening hours or on weekends. Also, some, probably many, physicians will reverse the long-term trend and once again make house calls, at least to treat the feeble elderly and others who are homebound. If there is a latent demand for such services and patients are able to pay for them, physicians are likely to respond.

The increasing supply of physicians is also likely to stimulate the rate at which new health care delivery systems are established and expand. A major explanation for the strikingly slow growth of prepaid delivery plans over the past decades has been the difficulty the plans encountered in attracting and retaining physicians and in working out effective relationships with specialists. Now that many more physicians are coming out of the pipeline and the number of attractive locations for starting practices has shrunk, prepaid group practice plans are encountering a better response to their recruitment and retention efforts.

The interaction between an increased supply of physicians and prepaid group practice plans can be extended to a much wider range of employment settings, from neighborhood health care clinics to state institutions. The much enlarged supply of physicians may further lead to a revision of state laws that have thus far interdicted the so-called corporate practice of medicine. If a growing number of young physicians encounter difficulties in establishing a private practice, they are more likely to look favorably on entrepreneurs who will underwrite new delivery systems that will offer them a reasonable environment for practice.

The growing numbers of specialists and primary care physicians entering practice in the years ahead point to a heightening of competition among members of the medical profession, competition that is likely to express itself in many guises, including fees, office hours, length of visits, feedback to patients, the use of procedures requiring out-of-pocket expenditures by patients, and still other aspects of practice.

The enlarged number of physicians is also likely to shift over the "power relations" in several critical areas between third-party payers and the medical profession. For example, physicians serving Medicare patients have had the option to accept or refuse assignments. Faced with mounting complaints from the elderly that they are forced to allocate an ever larger part of their income to pay for their unreimbursed health care costs, the federal government may conclude one of these days that the physician market has eased sufficiently for Medicare to change its reimbursement policies and require all physicians who treat Medicare patients to accept assignments.

Another possible consequence of the easing of the physician supply may be the elimination of the differential that currently exists between the fees paid to specialists and to nonspecialists for the same procedures. The procedure, rather than the credentials of the physician, will determine the rate of reimbursement.

The federal government reduced, in 1982, Medicare reimbursements for hospital-based physicians, particularly pathologists and radiologists, to conform with other physicians who receive 80 percent of their norm. It is possible that if the physician supply eases further, third-party payers will seek to eliminate contractual arrangements that award hospital-based physicians a percentage of the hospital's billings.

One of the dramatic changes in the post-World War II era has been the relocation of nurse education from the hospital, the historic training site for nurses, to collegiate settings where it has been integrated with the system of higher education. The combination of broadened career opportunities for college-educated women, higher rates of withdrawal from the nursing profession as a result of relatively low wages and strained working conditions, and a decline in the college-age cohort points to a relatively taut supply of nurses, particularly hospital nurses, for the remainder of this decade, especially if the economy makes a strong rebound.

There is no way to provide a summary overview of the several million additional health workers who receive training that ranges from a few weeks of on-the-job instruction to university preparation that involves the acquisition of a master's degree or a doctorate. The educational system proved highly responsive to the demand for more health care personnel during the decades of rapid expansion. With the deceleration or leveling off of this demand during the years ahead, there should be no problem in filling the available jobs. If anything, the opposite danger may arise. Should financial difficulties lead a significant number of health care institutions to close their doors, many medically trained workers may find themselves out of a job. We know that many hospital mergers are delayed or fail to materialize because of strong resistance based on a fear of redundancy.

A reasonable generalization for the years ahead is that with the possible, but by no means certain, exception of nurses, all major groups of health personnel are likely to confront a much changed employment scene. Good positions and high earnings will be more elusive than in the past several decades because of the altered balance between the number of providers and the demand for their services. In such an environment, the opportunities for new types of health care delivery systems will be greatly enhanced because the recruiters of medical specialists and supporting personnel will find themselves in a strong position. Nothing can contribute more to increasing competition in health care than a surplus of well-trained professionals.

HOSPITALS IN THE EARLY 1980s

If one were to identify a single area to illustrate the transformation of the U.S. medical care system in the period since World War II, it would be the hospital. The hospital has been the site of major advances in diagnosis and therapeutics, and the life-saving, pain-relieving, and restorative capabilities of modern medicine have been directly dependent on major improvements in hospital care.

The increased flow of payments to hospitals, stimulated initially by the growth of nonprofit and commercial insurance and later by government subsidization of care for the elderly and the poor, has enabled hospitals to increase and strengthen their professional and support staffs and to pay their staffs competitive salaries and wages, something that they had been unable to do previously.

Because most insurance policies in former years provided coverage only for inpatient services and not for ambulatory care (except in emergencies), a strong bias arose on the part of both physicians and patients to use, in fact overuse, the hospital as a treatment setting. As the issue of cost containment came to the fore, however, the control of hospital costs came to occupy center stage.

Every study of the comparative costs of fee-for-service practice versus prepaid delivery plans revealed that, after adjusting for differences in the age and other characteristics of patients in the two systems, prepaid delivery plans had substantially lower hospital utilization rates. The inference drawn from these studies was that an integrated system of ambulatory and inpatient care could help to reduce costly hospital admissions.

Reinforcement for this conclusion came when Blue Cross Plans and commercial insurance carriers began to relax their long-term resistance to providing coverage for ambulatory care. Although insurance carriers remained wary of including a broad range of ambulatory benefits in their policies, they saw gains in covering such services when they were linked to potential or actual hospital admission, such as preadmission diagnostic tests, emergency room care, or post-hospital treatment.

In the early 1970s, John Knowles, who was at the time director of the Massachusetts General Hospital, forecast that per diem charges in teaching hospitals might before long reach $350 or even $500. Almost no one gave his forecast credence. But the implausible has now become reality. To complicate matters, the financing of other elements of the health care system has also come under pressure: the tightening of governmental allocations for health care for the elderly and the poor; reduced federal support of medical education and research; high interest rates and the growing burden of debt incurred by hospitals in previous years, which has reduced their future ability to borrow in the capital markets; severe cash flow problems that an increasing number of hospitals are experiencing as a result of delays in payments by reimbursers; and the growing volume of "unpaid bills" resulting from the tightening of Medicaid coverage and the loss of insurance that accompanies high and prolonged unemployment. Large municipal and nonprofit hospitals located in the inner city close to concentrations of poor people are under the most severe financial pressure.

Because of the steady advances in sophisticated medical technology and procedures, the number of employees per 100 patients in short-term hospitals rose rapidly from 226 in 1960 to 370 in the late 1970s. About 30 percent of the rise in hospital costs is ascribed to the effects of technology, over 60 percent reflects inflation, and only 7 percent reflects gains in population.

The last decade has seen the onset of important changes in the structure and operations of hospitals as they enter a period of no growth or possible slow decline. The backbone of the short-term hospital system has long been the nonprofit community institution, which has accounted for over two-thirds of all acute care beds. The nonprofits still dominate this sector, but in the last decade proprietary institutions have grown substantially: from 53,000 beds in 1970 to 83,000 in 1979, or some 56 percent. State and local government facilities continue to be the second largest component of the short-term hospital system, accounting for slightly more than one out of every five beds.

Among the "external" forces that are beginning to encourage change in the ways in which hospitals perceive and pursue their mission are the increases in the supply of physicians, the growth of HMOs, initiatives by the federal government to explore alternatives to Medicare and Medicaid, prudent purchasing by third-party payers, a search to remove at least some of the costs of graduate medical education from payment for hospitalized patients, pressures on communities to pay for the hospital expenses of the near-poor that are no longer covered by government, curtailment of excess hospital beds, opportunities for hospitals to broaden the scope of services that they provide through the establishment or expansion of home health care programs, medical supervision of nursing homes, and similar community-based activities. These suggest early and substantial changes in the status quo, a number of which are assessed below.

Recent developments suggest that proprietary hospitals, particularly those that are part of a chain, are able to profit from economies of scale in the purchase of capital equipment and disposables. More important, they are in a preferred position to take advantage of basic operating systems—financial, inventory control, personnel, billing—that the chain has developed and often brought to a high level of effectiveness. Furthermore, chains are in a better position to attract, train, and use competent managers who are able to advance from smaller to larger hospitals as they acquire knowledge and experience. But the key to the financial success of many proprietary hospitals appears to be their superior marketing, tight financial controls, responsiveness to consumer desires, and avoidance or minimization of unprofitable types of activities, such as the training of residents and the operation of outpatient departments.

There is scattered evidence that the growth of proprietary chains may be speeded by local governments looking for an opportunity to withdraw from hospital operations in order to avoid the open-ended budgetary commitments that they confront in a period when the federal and state governments give every indication of reducing entitlement rolls and reimbursements. Although some city and county commissioners may succeed in transferring their hospital to a proprietary chain, it is unlikely, however, that large public hospitals in major metropolitan areas will disappear.

As important as proprietary and municipal hospitals are in selected locations, and allowing for the further growth of the proprietary sector, any serious discussion about hospitals in the 1980s must focus on the nonprofit institution, both the small community hospital and the large teaching hospital, which may be freestanding or one unit of a multihospital chain. These institutions dominate the acute care scene. How will changing forces, both internal and external, affect them and in what ways are they likely to react to ensure their survival and well-being?

Any attempt to answer this question must start with the basic premise that community hospitals, except for the largest medical centers, depend heavily on their ability to draw patients from their immediate environment. Their success in keeping their beds filled depends in turn on population trends in their neighborhood, the number of their competitors, their own professional and financial strengths, and underlying changes with respect to hospitalization.

It is reasonably certain that the combination of cost containment pressures, more physicians, slowed population growth, cutbacks in government financing of health care, high interest rates, and heavy indebtedness will place many hospitals in an exposed position. The last years have seen the beginning of a movement toward merger, conversion, and closure among hospitals that lack endowment funds to fall back on, face delays in payment by reimbursing agents, and are experiencing a decline in their bed occupancy. Their choice has been a simple one: to close or to merge. The power of the marketplace cannot be ignored. At some point, an institution that runs out of cash and can no longer borrow has lost its independence.

Among the survivors, what will the better-managed, financially stronger institutions do to ensure their long-term survival and well-being in an increasingly difficult environment? Large teaching hospitals in different parts of the country have begun to establish satellites, clinics, or affiliations with small hospitals for the purpose of assuring an adequate flow of patients to their institution. In other cases, referral agreements have been made with groups of independent medical practitioners to achieve the same goal: a steady flow of patients so that the hospital's occupancy rate remains above the break-even point.

Some larger hospitals are also entering into arrangements with HMOs, individual practice associations, and other types of health delivery plans. Hospitals offer office space, staff appointments, educational benefits, and volume discounts for inpatient care in return for an agreement by the physicians to admit all or most of their patients to the sponsoring hospital.

A second approach can best be described by the term "diversification." A hospital that previously limited its activities to treating inpatients and running an emergency room and outpatient clinics decides to broaden the range of health care services that it provides. Such expansion may call for the construction of a major adjunct facility for fee-for-service ambulatory care, initiation of a home health care program, development of preventive health care services for the work force of nearby industrial plants, and, even farther afield, ownership and operation of a health spa or the provision of physician services to a group of nursing homes.

Hospitals that face an uncertain environment but are not in a position to pursue diversification in health care services or to pursue other profit-making ventures may seek to affiliate with a hospital chain that offers them the prospect of benefiting from economies of scale and better access to the capital markets, and at the same time, allows them sufficient scope to command their own destiny.

It would be naive to assume that aggressive marketing, diversification, establishment of profit-making enterprises, or membership in a hospital chain will guarantee the future of every hospital in the adverse economic environment that lies ahead. The odds are strong that the 1980s will see a considerable reduction in the number of nonprofit hospitals, a diversification in the health care activities that surviving hospitals will engage in, and the growth of hospital chains.

If the federal government succeeds in restructuring Medicaid and Medicare through the introduction of vouchers or other means; if state legislators decide that the time has come to reduce enrollments in medical schools; if the specialty societies curtail residency training programs; if the exacerbating conflicts between nurses and hospitals are not moderated; if prepaid group practice plans experience a rapid rate of growth—if all or many of these developments occur in the years ahead, the pressures for a radical restructuring of the hospital sector will be that much greater. The resulting pattern of change will be revealed only with the passage of time. Nevertheless, it is safe to assume that even with less severe pressures, the hospital sector in 1990 will differ in many ways from that of today.

THE CHANGING HEALTH CARE MARKET

During the years of expansion, the ability of hospitals, primarily nonprofit institutions, to obtain the required additional resources depended on the fundamental willingness of the American people to meet the steadily rising costs of hospital care. They were enabled to do so by the vast expansion of insurance and other prepayment mechanisms and the decision of government to underwrite the costs of care for the elderly and the poor. Access of hospitals to the private capital markets for borrowing, usually via tax-exempt bonds repayable out of depreciation accounts, also helped to fuel the expansionary cycle.

The willingness of third-party payers, both insurance and government, to reimburse hospitals on the basis of their charges or their costs was another powerful stimulus, since most trustees and administrators saw little danger in increasing their expenditures to maintain their institution's primacy. Indeed, short-term hospitals, whose expenditures increased from just over $2.1 billion in 1950 to $66.2 billion in 1979, demonstrated a marked adaptability to the new opportunities provided by the advances in medicine, new sources of financing, and clear signals from middle-class America that wanted the benefits of improved hospital care to be available not only for themselves, but for all members of the community including the poor.

If this reconstruction of the long cycle of expansion of hospital care is fairly straightforward, the nursing home tale reveals a more checkered development for several reasons, chiefly the fact that its linkage to health care is not nearly so direct or unequivocal. In 1950, nursing home care represented about 1.5 percent of all national health expenditures, a measure of its insignificant role in the system. By 1980, however, it accounted for 8.4 percent of a vastly enlarged total outlay, reflecting a major absolute and relative increase.

Beginning in the early 1970s, when changed federal regulations permitted the use of Medicaid funds to pay for the care of indigent patients in intermediate care facilities, nursing homes grew rapidly. Today, approximately half of all nursing home expenditures are covered by Medicaid, mostly for the impoverished feeble elderly who require personal care. Although a minority of nursing home patients have recurrent need for skilled nursing and physician services, the majority require assistance primarily with such functions as walking, feeding, and toileting. The line between health care and these basic "maintenance" supports is not well defined. The fact, however, is that nursing homes characteristically devote most of their efforts to providing the latter, not the former. Paradoxically, this single fastest growing component of health care in the last three decades is only tangentially related to medical intervention and the amelioration or cure of disability or illness.

In contrast to the relative rise in hospital and nursing home expenditures, payments for physician services declined from 21.7 percent of all national health expenditures in 1950 to 18.9 percent in 1980. Notwithstanding this relative decline, expenditures per capita for physician services rose from under $18 in 1950, to $43 in 1965, to $113 a decade later, to over $201 in 1980—overall an elevenfold increase.

This large and sustained increase (unadjusted for inflation) reflects several major influences. First, the significant, if delayed, increase in the number of physicians enabled more people to obtain services. There was a substantial rise in the number of physician visits per person per year, particularly in the case of the poor, who averaged 3.9 visits in 1964 and 5.6 in 1978. A related measure is the proportion of the population that did not visit a physician during the preceding two years. Among the poor, there was a decline from 28 percent to 14 percent; among the nonpoor, from 18 percent to 13 percent.

Another factor worth noting is the "monetarization" of all medical services that followed the passage of Medicare and Medicaid. This meant that physicians no longer treated sizable numbers of patients free or for less than their customary charge. Further, the rise in office expenses, including malpractice insurance, and the growth of "defensive medicine" contributed to an escalation of fees. Physicians were also able to treat more patients and to increase their earnings by making greater use of the hospital as a treatment setting.

Looking back over this thirty-year span, the key transformations in the operation of the health care market have been the broadened access of all income groups to physicians and hospitals, the growing dominance of the hospital in the delivery of sophisticated medical services, the growth of nursing home care, and the large-scale flow of new funds into health care via insurance and governmental expenditures.

No less impressive are the continuities in the structure and operations of the health care system. Most physicians continue to practice medicine on a fee-for-service basis, many as solo practitioners, a growing number as members of small or large specialty or multispecialty groups. Most hospital care continues to be provided by nonprofit institutions that operate independently under the control of a board of trustees who represent the philanthropic and business leadership in the community.

Although health care expenditures via insurance increased during these three decades from $1 billion to over $60 billion and governmental outlays from $2.4 billion to $104 billion, neither of these payers has exercised much influence on how the principal providers—physicians, hospitals, and nursing homes—have conducted their operations. One can go a step further and say that the nation's employers and the unions that have negotiated group health coverage for the work force have concerned themselves more with the cost and range of health benefits offered by the carriers than with the ways in which their premium dollars are spent.

Two generalizations can be derived from this retrospective. First, once the flow of new dollars was assured, the health care system demonstrated substantial flexibility in expanding the range and depth of health care services it provided to the American people. Second, a remarkable stability prevailed in both the basic pattern of fee-for-service practice and the leadership role of the nonprofit hospital. Together these have continued to dominate the U.S. health care system.

With this backward perspective in mind, we can anticipate the decade ahead when many of the critical elements are likely to undergo rapid change. A deceleration in the growth of the demand for health care can be expected even in the absence of significant constrictions in financing. Most Americans have now gained access to the health care system and the rate of population growth is slowing. Countervailing influences are the steadily growing number of older people who are heavy users of health care and the expanding boundaries of medicine that recently have begun to stress preventive and rehabilitative care.

In the years ahead, an increasing number of young physicians will be more receptive to alternative modes of practice, to accepting a salaried position or joining the staff of a prepaid plan. Faced with the alternative of spending years in building a practice or in earning a share in a partnership, many young physicians will opt for a secure place on an institution's staff or employment in a prepaid plan.

In turn, the receptivity of a larger number of physicians to such positions will stimulate the development of new delivery systems that have been retarded in the past by difficulties in recruitment. Hospitals, hospital chains, insurance carriers, and other entrepreneurial enterprises with capital resources at their command will encounter less difficulty in acquiring the professional personnel they need to establish or expand alternatives to the dominant pattern of fee-for-service health care delivery.

Turning to the hospital sector, there has been a decline in the total number of days of care that hospitals provide. To make matters worse, third parties that reimburse for over 90 percent of all hospital outlays are increasingly concerned with the charges or costs that they are required to cover. The federal government, for instance, has been cutting back on the amount of reimbursable overhead costs of hospitals that it is willing to cover for Medicare and Medicaid patients. As a consequence, hospital administrators have had to load these and other uncovered costs onto the rates they charge commercial carriers and self-pay patients. Compounding these difficulties, many hospitals find themselves in a serious cash bind because of the slowness with which they are being reimbursed.

Looking ahead to the remainder of this decade, one sees intensified pressures in the hospital market resulting from weakened demand, tighter reimbursements, and greater competition from for-profit chains. If interest rates remain high, hospitals that must borrow capital for plant improvement will be particularly vulnerable. The odds are that many will not be deemed creditworthy and will be forced to merge to survive. A considerable number will not find a partner and will go under.

The turmoil in the hospital market will be exacerbated by the growing trend of physicians to treat patients in an ambulatory setting. This shift reflects multiple pressures but none more potent than the concern of physicians to protect their incomes. Third-party payers intent on reducing their outlays believe that one way to accomplish this is to encourage the treatment of patients in an ambulatory setting. Improvements in medical technology make it possible for many physicians to undertake in the office elaborate diagnostic procedures that formerly required a hospital setting. Surgeons now recognize that many procedures can be performed as satisfactorily in an ambulatory setting as in the hospital. But the probability that this withdrawal from the hospital will gain momentum rests chiefly on the realization by physicians that the best strategy to protect their share of health dollars is to slow the flow of patients into the high-cost environment of the hospital.

It would be wrong, however, to assume that the nonprofit hospital will be powerless to protect itself against the threats posed both by for-profit institutions and by the much enlarged supply of physicians. The modern well-equipped, well-staffed, short-term hospital represents the strongest component of the entire health care system. It is able to provide more and better care than any other element. It has a preferred relation to the community, having attracted and retained the loyalty of key leaders who are concerned for its survival. It is likely to have on its staff many of the most respected members of the medical profession. With annual revenues in the tens of millions, and in the case of the largest teaching hospitals, hundreds of millions, many nonprofit institutions are in a strong, not weak, market position.

What they cannot do is to stand still and expect to operate in 1990 as they operated in the 1970s. But there are signs that the more aggressive and better managed have begun to alter their operations to adjust to the changing market. These changes cover a wide front: organization, management, financing, marketing, and product mix.

The increases in physician supply that place many hospitals at risk because of the potential competition from outpatient practice by generalists and specialists will also make it easier for hospitals to recruit salaried staff. This in turn will permit them to expand the range of services that they provide and broaden the markets that they serve.

It is difficult to predict clearly how the better-managed and presumably stronger hospitals will respond to the changed market and the intensified competition that they will encounter. Early responses are already under way; many others are still beyond the horizon.

PRESSURE POINTS AND CHOICES

Without question, the increasingly frantic search of state and federal legislators to narrow the gap between their expenditures and revenues represents the most important pressure point affecting the health care system but it is by no means the only one. Even a short list must include the worsening financial outlook for the hospital system in a period of slow growth in future demand and heightened concern with cost containment. These pressure points involve both current operations and access to capital funds for modernization and improvement.

The purchasers of insurance—employers and labor—and the insurance carriers themselves—commercial companies and Blue Cross and Blue Shield Plans—comprise another pressure point. Until the last few years, the insurance mechanism operated relatively smoothly as purchasers sought more and better coverage. Carriers designed packages that were responsive to the market; major medical insurance is a case in point. The carriers in turn had relatively little difficulty securing the premium increases they needed to cover the costs of the improved policies that consumers demanded. But of late consumer resistance is coming to the fore. Both employers and the representatives of labor have become aware that health care benefits are commanding an ever larger share of their fringe benefits package, and in many instances the higher costs are not reflected in broadened benefits, but represent additional outlays to cover steep annual increases in the cost of health care.

The carriers are also under pressure because they have limited themselves largely to the role of reimbursing providers for the services they render, based on the provider's costs or charges. The carriers have made relatively little use of their potential leverage to exercise a restraining influence on costs.

Several powerful forces at work suggest that young physicians entering practice may represent another major pressure point. First, the rise in the ratio of physicians to population coinciding with strenuous efforts on the part of government and insurers to contain the rate of increase in outlays for health care will generate new tensions, particularly between physicians and hospitals, as to where and how patients are to be treated.

It is more than a decade ago since Dr. James Shannon, then head of the National Institutes of Health, testified before a congressional committee that as the pressures mounted for government to allocate even larger sums to finance medical service programs, there was a danger that the frontiers of medicine—education, research, and development—would be underfunded. Although the last years have confronted the academic health centers (the medical and health professional schools and their principal teaching hospitals) with shrinking resources, the outlook is likely to deteriorate further.

It is no accident that these pressure points represent key elements in the financing-provider structure: government, hospitals, insurers, physicians, and academic health centers. But these critical producer elements, important as they are, exist and grow only to the extent that they are responsive to the demands and needs of the paying and voting public that are the beneficiaries of an expanded and improved level of health care services. Hence, changes in the attitudes and behavior of the American public toward health care must be viewed as another pressure point, possibly the most important of all.

The early efforts of legislators to slow the rise in health care costs by cutting the numbers on entitlement rolls and reducing benefits, the agitation in Washington aimed at providing more scope for competitive forces, and the active interest of business and labor in health care costs are indicative of the growing concern and need of the American public to reassess both sides of the health equation. It can no longer focus exclusively on the expansion of desirable health care goals but must also consider the costs of such expansion.

To appreciate the choices we face requires a broader understanding of the ways in which the extant system is structured and operates. Such an analysis will help to identify the levers that can operate on the pressure points that have been identified. The dominant characteristics of the U.S. health care system that must be considered include:

- substantial variation in the patterns of health care utilization within and among different areas of the country, which reflect the public's preferences, resource availability, and professional practice
- the division of responsibility between different levels of government and the private sector to establish and control sta dards of performance, with physicians in the leading position to define and enforce such standards
- the scope for the "shifting" of charges and revenues among the three principal funding sources—consumers, insurers, and government—or when one of the funding sources reduces its level of effort
- the relative weakness of market forces to influence demand and price because of the dominant role of the physician in determining the range of required services, the importance of third-party payers, and the societal preference, if not commitment, to provide access to all irrespective of their ability to pay
- the role of academic health centers in shaping the values and behavior of future physicians and the continued dependence of the medical care system on these centers for innovation
- the public's overall satisfaction with the health care system as it currently operates except for restiveness about rising costs
- the difficulties in a mixed public-private system of improving existing mechanisms or introducing new ones that will contribute to the more efficient use of resources

For schematic purposes, one can distinguish five policy positions with respect to restructuring the health care system and altering its operations:

- maintenance of the status quo
- government cutbacks
- prospective hospital budgeting
- competition
- institutional and community reforms

The critical questions that need to be raised and answered are whether and to what extent the foregoing basic policy orientations appear to be responsive to the pressure points that have been identified. Given the sizable gap between emerging policy and pressure points, analysis reveals serious gaps in policy.

Although many of the key providers—physicians, hospitals, and nursing homes—would generally prefer to see the maintenance of the status quo (and in this they would be joined by insurance companies, academic health centers, and most of the public), there is little prospect that such aspirations will be realized in view of the budgetary pressures confronting the federal and state governments. But there are other important reasons why a policy favoring the status quo would fail. We have noted the large additions to the physician supply and the prospective leveling off of the growth of the hospital industry. These two developments are certain, sooner rather than later, to introduce significant alterations in the role of the two key provider groups. In short, the one reasonably certain conclusion is that a policy oriented to the status quo, that is congenial to most of the interested parties, will founder on the hard reality of an insufficient flow of funds into the system, particularly from the largest source, government.

There is another reason why a policy to maintain the status quo cannot succeed. An increasing number of purchasers of care, in particular business, labor, and organized consumer groups, are coming to believe that the extant system of delivering health care should be rationalized to a point where it produces the present level of service for a lower total cost. As this conviction intensifies, it will encourage purchasers to explore new approaches.

The second policy, government cutbacks of health expenditures, is clearly gaining momentum. Federal actions in 1982 saw modest reductions in Medicare reimbursement via reduced payments for ancillary services, nursing care, and fees for hospital-based physicians, and several state governments continued to tighten their rules governing Medicaid.

The 1984 federal budget proposals represent a stronger move in the direction of controlling future expenditures, particularly for Medicare. The administration's proposals include requiring beneficiaries to make copayments for hospital stays between the second and 59th days, increased premium payments by persons enrolled in supplemental medical insurance, a cap on deductible health insurance premiums paid for by employers, and a freeze on physician fees. The Congressional Budget Office estimated that for the years 1984–1988, the combined savings of the President's plan would amount to $29 billion. Congress legislated new savings in June 1984 but less drastic than the Administration had proposed.

One must also take note of parallel actions by state and local governments to restrain or even reduce future outlays for health care. Many states have recently cut back on Medicaid eligibility and on service coverage, placing a limit in some cases on the number of days of acute hospital care that they will reimburse. There is also mounting evidence that many hard-pressed county and local governments are seeking to close down or at least shrink their tax-supported hospitals.

The third policy focuses on prospective budgeting, which is predicated on informing hospitals in advance of the rate at which they will be reimbursed for the care of patients. Several states, particularly New York and Maryland, have resorted to prospective budgeting for the better part of a decade. Recent studies suggest that increases in these states' hospital costs have been slowed, though frequently with dysfunctional concomitants such as forcing some hospitals to deplete their endowments and forcing others into bankruptcy.

In 1982, the federal government granted both Massachusetts and New York a Medicare waiver that will permit them for the first time to regulate the rates that hospitals charge different groups of patients, thereby placing a limit on cross-subsidization as well as providing a pool of money to cover charity care and bad debts.

The federal government has legislated a system of prospective reimbursement for Medicare patients based on diagnosis-related groups (DRGs), which went into effect in October 1983. A DRG system has had a field run in New Jersey, but has not yet yielded definitive findings.

It would be a serious error to assume, however, that prospective budgeting provides an easy answer to the twin challenges of setting limits on future government outlays and of slowing the rise in hospital costs. The more dynamic the health care market as reflected in changes in hospital capacity, patient admissions, technological advances, and other factors, the greater the difficulty of using the experience of the past as a basis for determining an institution's expenditures and revenues in the future. Such difficulties notwithstanding, prospective budgeting offers government one possible escape from its present untenable position of continuing open-ended commitments to cover hospital costs for the large proportion of the population for which it is responsible.

The fourth policy approach to contain health care prices—the procompetition approach—has gained a number of adherents in Congress, who, pressed by their constituents to oppose greater regulation and confronting large budgetary deficits, are seeking a way out of ever-increasing government expenditures for health care.

There are two major versions of the procompetition approach, one that looks to "fair competition," as Enthoven has proposed, and the other the creation of Representatives Gephardt and Stockman (when the latter sat in the House of Representatives), which looks to an almost total reliance on market forces and the reduction of the federal government's health care role to a minimum. These are worth inspecting, even if neither is likely to provide the basis for new legislation. The ideas that they advance continue to some degree to inform the debate.

The objectives of the procompetition approach are to force individual consumers to play a more active role in determining their health care expenditures by limiting the value of tax-exempt health benefits that they can receive from their employers; to encourage them to choose among competing types of health insurance or provider plans, even to the extent of offering them a rebate if they choose a less costly plan; and to stimulate providers to develop alternatives to the dominant fee-for-service system of practice. If physicians and hospitals have to compete more intensively for patients on the basis of price, advocates of competition are certain that costs will rise more slowly.

In the Gephardt-Stockman version, health care consumers would have even greater freedom. Employers would no longer offer employees a choice of plans. Workers would simply be given vouchers of a specified value with which to search the market, and then select and purchase such coverage as best fits their needs.

The influence of alternative delivery systems on cost containment is uncertain. In California, strong HMOs have operated alongside fee-for-service practice for several decades. So too in Washington, D.C., and more recently in the Twin Cities. Theory notwithstanding, it is not clear that such competition has had a significant effect on cost containment.

There are additional reasons to question whether federal legislative action that is strongly supportive of increased competition in health care delivery would yield the benefits that its supporters anticipate. The following are some of the reasons for caution:

- Selling and administrative costs could skyrocket.
- The consumer is sometimes in a poor position to judge what is offered, especially as it relates to complex coverage for health care services.
- The problem of protecting against adverse selection could make coverage increasingly expensive for those most in need.
- The elimination of controls over new construction could result in excessive hospital capacity followed by institutional closures that would find neighborhoods and communities first overbedded and then underbedded.

There are several additional reasons to question the putative gains from the procompetition approach, including the questionable power of the federal government to establish insurance rates that take account of regional variations in costs, the serious threat to academic health centers and their principal affiliates from a no-holds-barred form of competition based on price, the uncertainty that will be introduced into the physician-patient relationship once price becomes a dominant consideration, and the loss of current efficiencies under the most extreme Gephardt-Stockman proposal that would eliminate the group policies that currently dominate the market.

These concerns do not imply that all efforts to stimulate additional competition would be dysfunctional. Far from it. The last decade has witnessed the growth of for-profit hospitals and hospital chains. Nursing homes are dominated by for-profit enterprises. The growing home health care field is also seeing for-profit enterprises increasing their share of the market. HMOs and other types of prepayment plans are growing, if at a slower pace than many would wish, and several major insurance companies have entered the field and are willing to provide the required capital to establish and expand prepaid delivery plans. Nonprofit hospitals, facing a slower growth in revenues and an intensified struggle for patients, are seeking new market opportunities that are leading them to diversify their operations. And there are many signs that with the rapid growth in the number of physicians in active practice, competition for patients is intensifying, which in time should contain somewhat the cost of a patient visit.

The federal government is exploring the introduction of a Medicare voucher system that the administration believes will encourage hospitals, physician groups, and prepayment plans to compete more aggressively on the basis of price for this strategically important sector of the health care market. A critical question is whether the elderly would gain or lose; currently the major coalitions of the elderly are strongly opposed to the proposal. It must also be noted that active antitrust enforcement has made it more difficult for providers to act collaboratively to influence the market to obtain above-average returns.

There is little support in theory or in historical experience for the belief that legislative action to impose competition as the guiding principle for the health care market could in fact succeed or that, if it did, the rise in total expenditures would be moderated. Indeed, the burden of the evidence suggests the opposite. However, one must quickly assert that even in the absence of such heroic legislation the health care market will undergo many changes that point to intensified competition among critical provider groups in the years ahead. The federal government, through its dominant role in the Medicare-Medicaid arena, could encourage these developments.

Although the administration has been slow to put forward a coherent proposal to increase competition in the health care market and Congress has demonstrated no inclination to take the lead, Arizona and California have moved aggressively to slow their outlays by forcing providers to bid for Medicaid patients. Both states award contracts for the care of Medicaid enrollees to hospitals and other provider institutions based on competitive bids. The California administrator stated that he hoped to save $200 million in the first year of operation. Even if this goal were realized, the net social cost might shave these savings to a greater or lesser extent, depending on how one counts the adverse effects on hospitals that lost out in the competition, the disturbance in physician-patient relations, and the difficulties of avoiding erosion in the quality of care provided Medicaid beneficiaries.

This preferred provider organization (PPO) approach to containing health care costs is not limited to state initiatives. Large employers, sometimes on their own and sometimes as members of business coalitions, are pressing hospitals in their communities for significant discounts based on the volume of their business and on the reliability and speed of their payments. Insurance plans are increasingly offering inducements to their policyholders to select a particular provider or a particular setting (ambulatory) for treatment. In the face of a growing number of physicians and new modes of delivering care, the PPO initiative is likely to develop considerable momentum.

The fifth and final approach to health care policy suggested herein is subsumed under the rubric of institutional and community reforms. The heart of this approach is that economies and efficiencies can be achieved primarily through improved control over the flow of resources into the system and corresponding efforts to improve the utilization of the resources that are available.

Many health care analysts are concerned that various parts of the country are seriously overbedded. The authors of the Graduate Medical Education National Advisory Committee report are convinced that the country faces an oversupply of physicians beyond the numbers needed to provide a satisfactory level of care to the entire population. Moreover, the burden of professional opinion holds that there are significant gains to be achieved in resource utilization by shifting a substantial proportion of patient treatment from inpatient to ambulatory care settings. The leadership of coalitions of the elderly and gerontologists favor increased opportunities for care at home and in the community in preference to institutionalization. Many leaders of the medical profession are opposed to the uncritical use of high technology and invasive procedures in the treatment of a substantial number of patients for whom less intensive interventions would be preferable, in terms both of desired outcomes and of cost.

If the essence of cost containment is, in fact, linked to a reduction in the inflow of resources, material and human, to the use of optimal settings for care, to improved coordination among the various settings from tertiary care centers to home health care, and to the selection of appropriate treatment modalities, then clearly there is no possible way for sweeping new legislation or other radical societal interventions to assure an appropriate level of resources and their more efficient use.

Such gains can be accomplished only by changes in the educational environments where future physicians are trained, in the treatment settings where health care services are provided, and in improved linkages within the spectrum of health care institutions. There is no way for states and localities to escape the challenge of estimating what they must spend in resource development to provide the appropriate infrastructure for an acceptable level of health care to their population, and for community leaders working with hospitals and health professionals to develop, on a local and regional basis, improved linkages among provider institutions to assure the effective use of resources.

The cynic could respond that an approach based on state, regional, and community action is bound to fail because the most powerful interest groups will prevent reforms that threaten their position. It is true that medical schools, large hospitals, and organized physician groups would prefer not to change. Clearly, in a society such as ours that is dominated by interest groups, the most potent units will fight the hardest not to give up power or income. But that does not mean that they will always be able to prevent sensible and sound reforms. The best way to assure against such obstruction is for those who control the purse in the public and private sectors—government, insurance, philanthropy, business, and labor—to become informed and participate actively in efforts to rationalize and improve the system. The task will not be easy, but in the absence of a preferred alternative this appears to be the best way to proceed.

The thrust of the foregoing has been to emphasize that the status quo in the health care arena cannot be expected to continue unaltered; that governments will make increasing efforts to bring their health expenditures under control; that prospective budgeting for hospitals may prove a constructive next step; that the advocates of strong procompetition legislation have not confronted the complexities of their proposal but that, despite the likely refusal of Congress to act, greater competition will nonetheless characterize the future market for health care; and that providers, underwriters, and users of health resources, from state governments to local community leaders, with a concern for efficient health care must play a larger role in helping to determine the appropriate level of resources required and how resource utilization can be improved.

The maintenance of a dynamic health care system at a sustainable cost will require short- and long-term strategies to alter the behavior of the principal parties; the public that seeks care; health care providers, particularly physicians and hospitals; and the principal payers for care—the consumer, government, and insurers. There is much that they can do individually as well as much that requires collaborative action at the community level:

- The public needs to develop greater understanding of the limits of medical intervention to constrain demands that cannot be satisfied.
- Patients must assume greater responsibility for their health by adopting healthier life-styles and by seeking help early, at a time when their condition is more amenable to treatment and the prognosis more favorable.

- Financial and other incentives should be introduced to encourage providers to control their costs without depriving patients of access to treatment that promises substantial relief or cure.
- Physicians and patients must reach an understanding to limit the use of high-cost technology where the outcomes are questionable or the procedures are contraindicated, as in the case of certain moribund patients.
- Mechanisms should be devised to encourage the shifting of care from high cost to less costly settings, that is, from acute hospitals to ambulatory settings.
- It is axiomatic that all members of the community, irrespective of ability to pay, must have access to essential health care services through the use of tax dollars, supplemented, if necessary, by contributions from the private sector. This can be assured only by a concerned and dedicated community leadership that recognizes and acts to discharge its responsibility.
- Funding must be provided for an optimal number of academic health centers at a level that will enable them to continue to advance the frontiers of medical knowledge and research. In view of the potential surplus of physicians, consolidations and mergers in cities with multiple centers should be explored.
- A community instrumentality must be established that will elicit the ongoing participation of the leadership of the principal concerned groups—physicians, hospitals, insurers, business and labor, local and state governments, and consumers—each of which has an important stake in assuring that good health care is provided at a sustainable cost and that all have access to the system.

The thrust of the foregoing strategies is to accomplish several interrelated objectives:

- to encourage the leadership in each community to re ognize its obligation to become involved in improving health care delivery for all persons in their area
- to reduce the utilization of nonproductive high-cost medical care
- to modify the present patterns of care so that costs can be better controlled without compromising access or quality

In a democracy such as the United States with its local and regional differences, progress depends on understanding, leadership, and community action, particularly with respect to the delivery of professional services. This does not mean that action in the centers of governmental power, in Washington and in state capitals, is unimportant but only that federal and state policies can do little more than set the boundaries. What happens within these boundaries to improve the use of resources, to raise the quality of care, and to assure equity depends primarily on local leadership and community response. Our complex health care system is in need of constraint, but this goal must not be pursued so indiscriminately as to jeopardize the major accomplishment of the system: the delivery of a high level of care to most of the American people.

Significant improvement in health care delivery can never be achieved by the passage of laws such as procompetition or by sole recourse to an administrative device such as prospective budgeting. Significant improvement requires continuing adjustments in the use of resources informed by the lessons of experience.

PART II

The Mirage of Competition

Economists have little modesty. When they are asked, and sometimes on their own, they offer opinions on every conceivable subject from criminal justice to education, from atomic weapons to health care. For most of this century, they ignored health care in favor of more exciting subjects. But as health care came to consume 10 percent of the GNP and as the inflation of health care prices continues to outpace general inflation, it was inevitable that economists would be drawn to the subject.

The three chapters that comprise Part II focus on a single question. To what extent is the basic model of economics—the competitive market—useful in analyzing the operations of the U.S. health care system, and to what extent does it provide guidance for establishing public policy that aims to assure access, efficiency, and quality at a lower total social cost?

Chapter 5 confronts the issue head-on. It contends that many of the presumed gains from more competition may result in cost increases, not cost decreases. It further contends that the political support for many of the proposals, such as a ceiling on tax deductions for health insurance benefits or the organization of physicians into prepaid practice arrangements, is not widespread and is not likely to expand rapidly in the near and middle term. The chapter focuses on the proposal advanced by Alain Enthoven, who took the lead in advocating a competitive solution.

Chapter 6 reminds the reader that while most health economists use the competitive model, some economists, including Nobel Laureate Kenneth Arrow, long ago pointed out the inherent limitations of the market to deal effectively and efficiently with problems of health insurance, health personnel, and still other basics of health care delivery. In their attempt to find a simple solution, the enthusiasts for a competitive solution simply ignored Arrow's work, thereby setting the stage for a later confrontation with his earlier arguments. The new converts to a competitive solution might ignore Arrow but they do not thereby overcome his objections.

Because much of the debate in medical economics has taken place in professional journals which are not normally seen by the medical profession, Chapter 7 recapitulates the critical arguments for physicians; it points out that economists do not talk with one voice on the subject of competition. In fact, the chapter emphasizes the inevitable and persistent gaps between the assumptions of the theory and the realities of health care and concludes that the competitive solution is a grand illusion. The whole of Part II emphasizes that when important issues such as health care costs come on the nation's agenda, theory, facts, and preferences are commingled with the result that politics and policy become confused.

5

Competition and Cost Containment

Several years have passed since Professor Alain Enthoven of Stanford University described in nontechnical language the rationale of his Consumer Choice Health Plan (CCHP).[1] The proposal, developed initially at the request of Secretary Califano of the Department of Health, Education, and Welfare, failed to win the administration's support, but in the period since it began to circulate, it has won adherents in the Congress[2] and among businessmen and has informed a growing number of economists and other social scientists concerned with the formulation of public policy for health care and regulation.

With steadily rising health care expenditures,[3] and with widespread concern on the part of employers, labor, and other groups about the continuing escalation of costs, any plan that promises to contain these powerful trends and to do so by relying on the impersonal forces of the market rather than on more layers of bureaucracy is bound to attract supporters. The time has come to look more closely at what Enthoven and his associates are proposing, if only to deepen the level of analysis in the search for improved policy.

No matter how many serious questions may be raised about the CCHP and its several variants, it must be acknowledged that Enthoven, in developing his proposal, made an important contribution to improving the level of the dialogue, through sharpening the questions and focusing on the relation between market incentives and market behavior in pointing up policy alternatives.

Originally published as "The Competitive Solution: Two Views," *New England Journal of Medicine* 303:19 (1112–15), November 6, 1980. Reprinted by permission.

Oversimplified, his catena for reform contains the following elements:

- Congress should alter the tax laws so that a ceiling is placed on the total amount of health insurance premiums that employers may deduct as a business expense, as well as on the value of nontaxable benefits that employees may receive.
- Employers must offer their workers a choice of at least three different health insurance plans, all of which must meet minimal standards for coverage. An employee who chooses a plan costing less than the most expensive plan that the employer offers will be entitled to pocket the difference.
- To make consumers of health care more cost conscious at the point of use, the plans should rely on coinsurance or deductibles.
- Special provisions should be made for enrollment and health insurance coverage of people with low incomes.

The three key concepts are tax changes to equalize subsidies among competing plans; consumer choice among competing plans, with incentives for purchasers to select the less expensive; and copayments to discourage overuse by consumers at the point of seeking care. The potential of competition to contain health care costs must start with an assessment of the foregoing critical elements even if it must inevitably move beyond such an assessment to include institutional arrangements and political realities.

Enthoven and his colleagues are correct in contending that the federal tax provisions, which enable employers to deduct all their expenditures for health insurance on behalf of their work force and which in turn treat all benefits received by employees as nontaxable income, encourage overspending for health insurance. Recent estimates set these specific tax benefits at $9.6 billion. Still another important tax benefit, with an estimated annual cost to the United States Treasury of about $3.1 billion, reflects deductions from personal income tax liability of part of the premium costs of health insurance and out-of-pocket medical expenditures in excess of 5 percent of net income.[4]

Liberal tax benefits not only inflate total spending for health insurance but have the further dysfunctional effect of reducing any incentive on the part of the purchaser to undertake comparison shopping with the aim of selecting a less expensive rather than a more expensive plan.

A third inherent defect of the present health insurance market is the substantial, implicit subsidy provided to the more expensive plans when employers pay for the total premiums of alternative plans, irrespective of cost differentials. This practice surely hobbles the opportunities for low-cost plans to expand.

These three shortcomings—encouraging excessive spending for health insurance, removing the incentive for consumers to shop among competing plans, and subsidies for high-cost plans—cannot be viewed as minor defects unworthy of attention and correction. But the potential for successful intervention cannot be assumed; it must be carefully explored. Most societal arrangements leave a great deal to be desired. The challenge to the reformer is not only to specify what is malfunctioning but also to point to remedial action that will cost less than the prospective benefits.

In the light of this criterion, the major revision of the health benefits provisions of the federal tax code, as proposed by the advocates of competition, calls for critical review. First of all, it is well to recall that the expansion of benefits was the outgrowth of a process of collective bargaining (and when there was no union, management was influenced by union settlements) in which workers paid for an improved health care package through forgoing some wages or other benefits. The imposition by Congress of a ceiling on nontaxable health care benefits that would be far below the upper level of existing benefits would represent an arbitrary tax on the income of certain workers that would be hard to justify on grounds of equity or efficiency. For market competition advocates to support such a major intrusion of the federal government into collective bargaining is a reminder that reformers are no more immune than other groups to becoming enthralled with their own ideology.

There is another reason to look critically at the proposal to alter the federal tax laws so that competition among health care plans may be enhanced. The free market advocates largely disregard the extent to which hardheaded bargaining currently prevails among many well-matched buyers and sellers. A large number of unions and employers consult specialists to help choose among a variety of benefit packages and plans, and commercial insurance companies, the Blue Cross and Blue Shield plans, and health maintenance organizations are selling in the same market. Admittedly, the tax laws bias the behavior of both buyers and sellers in the direction that the CCHP has outlined—toward more expensive plans—but only up to a point. Both employers and unions are interested in stretching their dollars as far as possible. What is spent on health is not available for other desirable objectives. The tax provisions alter the shape of competition in the health care market, but they do not preclude its presence or growth.

I agree with Enthoven that if the tax subsidy for high-cost plans could be substantially reduced or eliminated and if employees could pocket the "savings" between a low-cost plan and the allowable ceiling underwritten by their employers, less expensive plans would be in a preferred position to compete and grow. But important issues remain. How fast would alternative delivery systems develop, and what are some of the likely consequences of their growth?

With regard to the speed with which new delivery systems would make their entrance, I believe that Enthoven has underestimated the barriers to their growth. Most physicians will continue to be hesitant to enter types of practice in which they are at serious financial risk and must conform closely to group standards. Moreover, the CCHP has provided only a few hints about ways of improving the integration of ambulatory care with hospital care and with care provided by other institutions. Enthoven was careful to avoid the oversimplification that health maintenance organizations alone hold promise of definitive gains in increasing the efficiency and reducing the cost of basic health care services. I believe that the growth of new systems for delivering care must overcome the deep resistance of physicians, other health providers, and consumers to relinquish any sizable part of their freedom of independent action.

The CCHP may be exaggerating the responsiveness of the market to the elimination of tax subsidies. There is little in recent experience to suggest that the consumer is guided in the purchase of professional services—educational, financial, legal, or architectural—primarily by considerations of price. Of course, price remains important, but so are convenience, quality, reliability, and other considerations.[5] The assumption that a public that reports general satisfaction with its regular source of health care will shift to another system of care even if it reduces total costs by 15 to 25 percent is problematic.[6]

Increased competition can do little by itself to constrain the rise in costs that reflects the public's determination to obtain access to the panoply of therapeutic services, ranging from sophisticated diagnostic tests to open-heart surgery. The CCHP does not specify what services must be covered or what may be omitted from approved plans so that they may compete. If these increased consumer demands are a major factor in increased costs, intensified competition may prove less effective in containing costs than its proponents anticipate.

The emphasis that the CCHP places on coinsurance and deductibles suggests that competition will need firm assistance from the consumer to slow, if not stop, the steady rise in costs. The advocates of competition want consumers to feel the pain of parting with their limited dollars at the moment of purchase, as a means of moderating demand for more numerous and more expensive services.

Here are a few challenges: The thirty-year effort to extend insurance coverage and to increase benefits has been aimed at reducing the risks to the consumer who is confronted with a medical emergency. Nevertheless, the consumer still pays 32 percent of the cost out-of-pocket.[7] The *Social Security Bulletin* has revealed that about two-thirds of all persons 65 or older carry supplementary private insurance for hospital care, over 55 percent carry supplementary insurance for services from a surgeon, and over 43 percent for in-hospital visits to a physician.[8]

The American consumer, irrespective of age, has repeatedly demonstrated a desire for first dollar coverage. This desire may make little sense to economists (myself included), but it is a fact that cannot be ignored. The situation of the American consumer is not unique; over the past fifteen years, the French government has attempted to impose universal cost sharing on French consumers by regulating the amount of supplementary coverage that could be offered, but these efforts have aroused widespread opposition and have failed.

Major medical insurance, the fastest growing type of health insurance other than dental insurance, is predicated on large deductibles in addition to a typical 20 percent coinsurance provision. An unsympathetic reading of the CCHP would suggest that the consumer should be discouraged from purchasing many services that the physician considers beneficial. I see little likelihood that the American public will adopt this approach to cost control.

Tax revision, consumer incentives to choose among competing plans, and coinsurance all have something in their favor as ways of increasing competition in health care delivery and of slowing the rise in health care costs. But for the reasons given above, I believe that the CCHP vastly overestimates the potential effectiveness of these remedies and vastly underestimates other factors influencing the steady rise in costs. A few observations on the realities of the health care system that have been ignored or underestimated by proponents of greater competition are necessary.

The CCHP recognizes several important roles for public policy: to define the elements that must be included in any competitively approved plan; to set rules governing enrollment; and to provid for coverage of the poor. But it is silent, or largely so, on such critical matters as the role of public policy in determining the number of students accepted in medical schools; the dominance of the voluntary sector in providing acute hospital care; excess bed capacity; public underwriting of certain treatments such as renal dialysis; the need for standards of quality assurance; and the urgent necessity to explore the integration of income, health, and welfare services for older persons, to reduce institutionalization.

Understandably, the advocates of competition might complain that the foregoing list of issues involving public interest only strengthens their contention about the desirability of shifting more responsibility for health care as quickly as possible to the market, to prevent the public authorities from being overwhelmed with challenges that they cannot possibly meet through regulation because of lack of time, talent, consensus, or money.

But the confrontation goes beyond those who favor more competition as the preferred approach to cost containment and those who reject it. The institutional elements identified above point to two inherent shortcomings in the position of the advocates of competition: the extent to which the preconditions for effective competition exist in the health care industry, and the extent to which costs are being driven by factors other than inefficiencies in the marketplace and undue reliance on third-party payers.

Consider the following: The private sector has never had more than a minor role in the construction and operation of hospitals. Even with recent expansion, profit-making hospitals control less than 10 percent of all acute care beds. Consider further that no producer enters a competitive market unless there is the prospect of profits, and that no producer who suffers repeated losses remains in that market. The provision of adequate capacity to meet the needs of the total population for hospital care can no more be relegated to the competitive market than can the adequate development and production of national weaponry; the record of repeated and large cost overruns in experiments with competitive bidding on weapons procurement contracts is testimony to the limitations of competition in ensuring a sufficient stream of public necessities.

At present, there is a consensus among experts that the nation has an excess of 100,000 to 150,000 acute care beds, the cost of which, no matter how calculated, comes to not less than several billion dollars a year.[9] There is no way—surely no direct way—of eliminating these excess beds, and it would take a bedrock faith in competition to let the market take over and do the elimination. There is nothing in the theory of competition to ensure that the resources required by the poor and the isolated for essential medical care will continue to be available. The recent closure of an increasing number of inner-city hospitals raises a warning that may not be disregarded.

Consider the supply of physicians, which will have expanded by about one-third at the end of the 1980s, when the American population will be increasing very slowly. Competition will unquestionably have an adverse effect on physicians' earnings.[10] But the total cost to society of such an increase in manpower, even if one does not accept uncritically the formula that physicians generate 70 percent of all health care costs, will be very large indeed.

Consider another example of the limitations of competition to control the factors underlying the rise in costs. Health care has been transformed during the past decades because of advances in research, development, and application, reflecting primarily cooperation among medical schools, teaching hospitals, and the pharmaceutical and equipment industries. Technology assessment may or may not be an effective method for controlling these costs, which reflect the growing capacity of the system to perform. But I see nothing except trouble ahead if the nation's teaching hospitals are forced to compete with community hospitals in providing routine services, since the former's per diem costs are one and one-half to two times as high as the latter's, as a result of their diverse output, which goes far beyond performing an appendectomy or hysterectomy and involves such critically important societal goals as training the next generation of physicians and adding to the pool of knowledge and technique. Enthoven appreciates this challenge, but the CCHP has not addressed it adequately.[11]

Despite its growing commitment to deregulation, the Carter administration did not sponsor the CCHP. Apparently the administration's principal objection was to the danger of adverse selection among competing health care delivery plans; the poor and the near poor might be left without satisfactory coverage. In addition, the administration saw little prospect of securing the passage of the CCHP since the plan involved such a radical interference with the collective bargaining process and an arbitrary reduction in worker benefits. I approve of this decision based on equity, Realpolitik, or both.

This brief analysis has sought to meet the CCHP on its own ground. On the basis of such a reconsideration, I conclude that the combined force of reduced tax benefits, increased consumer incentives to shop for more cost-efficient plans, and greater reliance on coinsurance would not lead to a substantial increase in cost-efficient delivery systems and that the multiplication of such delivery systems would not slow the expansion of health care costs in a fashion that would be acceptable to the American people. The public wants improved, not reduced, access to essential health care, and it wants to accelerate, not slow down, the progress of medical science.

We are indebted to Enthoven for outlining a potent alternative. Although it has been rejected for what appear to be good and sufficient reasons and the mixed system in which the market and social pressure share responsibility has been retained, we are still in his debt for forcing us to think more deeply and more critically about the shortcomings of the existing system. This critical thinking gives us another opportunity to advance.

6

Competition:
Policy or Fantasy?

For the better part of three-quarters of a century social reformers sought to persuade the American people that national health insurance (NHI) was the only practical answer to providing universal access to health care. Around the time of World War I, even the American Medical Association favored the enactment of NHI, but within a few years it retreated and assumed leadership of the opposition.

After a long journey in the wilderness, the reformers scored their first success in 1965 with the passage of Medicare and looked forward to final victory in a two-stage advance: the proximate passage of insurance for mothers and children to be followed by coverage for other adults.

Even in the absence of coverage for mothers and children, the chairman of the Ways and Means Committee of the House of Representatives, Representative Al Ullman, prophesied in the spring of 1976 that the long-delayed victory was at hand: Congress would pass NHI and President Ford would be reluctant to veto it in the face of the approaching election.

Ullman proved to be a poor prophet. Congress never came close to passing NHI. What is more, six years later, public opinion polls now find that only one out of every ten respondents places NHI high on his or her list of priorities. This encapsulated account of the natural history of NHI should serve as a reminder that the current excitement about imminent congressional action to legislate competition into health care may yet turn out to be of passing, not permanent, interest.

Irrespective of the eventual outcome the arguments advanced by the proponents of competition warrant close scrutiny. The trend toward ever

Originally published as "Procompetition in Health Care: Policy or Fantasy?," *Milbank Memorial Fund Quarterly/Health and Society* 60:3(386–98), Summer, 1982. Reprinted by permission.

higher health care expenditures, considerably in excess of the rate of inflation, appears to many to make the competition proposal the only game in town.

THE COMPETITIVE STRATEGY

The principal building blocks in the competitive solution are:

- Increased choice to consumers at the point when they purchase health insurance or select a prepaid health delivery plan. Such a broadening of options can be assured by legislative mandate that 1) requires each employer to offer his employees a choice of at least three plans, 2) establishes a monetary incentive for the consumer to select a less costly plan, and 3) takes the employer out of the insurance transaction completely other than to provide a "health care contribution" for each employee with which to shop the market.
- A ceiling on the maximum amount of tax-free health benefits that the employer could cover. If the employer agrees to a plan with a higher premium, both outlays and benefits received by employees above the maximum allowable figure would be subject to tax.
- Higher deductibles and more copayments, usually with a tradeoff in the form of coverage for catastrophic expenditures after a family has incurred large out-of-pocket expenses (in the range of $2,500 to $3,500) during the course of the year.
- A Medicare voucher, set at 95 percent of average adjusted per capita cost and indexed for inflation, to broaden the choice of the elderly. It would be offered initially on a voluntary basis.
- Reduction and elimination of many regulatory approaches to health care cost containment, extending even to preemption by the federal government of state regulation of insurers.
- New forms of prepaid health care delivery that will help to control costs, encouraged by the foregoing reforms.

KENNETH ARROW REVISITED

Before looking more closely at the heart of the competitive proposals—enhanced consumer choice,[1] prudent purchasing of insurance,[2] limitation on tax benefits,[3] increased copayment,[4] Medicare vouchers,[5] less regulation,[6] and more prepaid provider plans[7]—one should review what the Nobel Laureate economist Kenneth Arrow (1963) wrote about competition in health care in his essay, "Uncertainty and the Welfare Economics of Medical Care."[8] Admittedly the passage of the intervening years has seen a great many changes in the health care system of the United States, not the least of which has been the introduction of Medicare and Medicaid. But our concern is less with institutional change and more with the theory of the health care marketplace which Arrow elaborated. Arrow's twelve principal arguments against the indiscriminate application of competitive criteria to assess the efficiency of the health care market may be summarized as follows:

- Insurance, the market's answer to risk, will always be less than perfect because health insurance will be unable to distinguish adequately among risks, especially between avoidable and unavoidable risks, and thus incentives to avoid losses will be diluted.
- In the face of uncertainty, information becomes a commodity but differs considerably from the usual marketability of commodities.
- Demand for health care is both irregular and unpredictable and medical services provide satisfaction only in the event of illness.
- The advice that the physician provides ought to be completely divorced from self-interest. Since the nature of the physician-patient relationship affects the quality of the medical care product, a pure cash nexus would be inadequate.
- In the face of product uncertainty, no patient ever experiences a sufficient number of trials to eliminate residual uncertainty.
- Price competition is frowned upon and physicians do not see themselves as maximizing profit. Nevertheless, the patient retains a freedom of choice that effects changes in the market, albeit slowly.
- Making tuition cover the full cost of medical education, as some free marketeers have suggested, will result in too few entrants.
- The availability of insurance increases the demand for medical care but the professional relationship between physician and patient limits the moral hazard.
- Large economies of scale in administrative costs point to the advantages of comprehensive plans, including a compulsory system.
- The preferred approach is for the maximum possible differentiation of risks, but there is a tendency to equalize rather than differentiate premiums which would not be the case if the market were genuinely competitive.
- Under ideal conditions, the patient could seek ins rance protection against a failure to benefit from medical care. The social obligation for the best in current practice is intrinsic to the commodity that the physician sells. Rigid entry requirements are designed to reduce uncertainty in the mind of the consumer as to the quality of the product.
- The failure of the market to insure against uncertainties has created many social institutions in which the usual assumptions about the market are to some extent contradicted.

Arrow's analysis warns against any simplistic projection of the competitive model onto health care because of many "imperfections" including, but not limited to, the following: the nature of the risk and the inability to insure fully against it; the imbalance between the information available to the buyers and the sellers of health care services; the desirability in the physician-patient relationship of minimizing the cash nexus; and the substantial economies of scale realized from large-scale insurance coverage.

COMPETITIVE THEORY: TWO READINGS

What can be learned from juxtaposing the schema advanced by the competition advocates and Arrow's critique of the limits of competition in health care? Once one recognizes the inherent limitations in sophistication of laymen with respect to medical care, the high costs of their acquiring information, and the inability to draw valid conclusions from their own experiences and exposures, the benefits of increased consumer choice become problematic. There may be little gain and conceivably considerable loss in encouraging consumers to shop for the least costly plan if one postulates that they are incapable of drawing valid conclusions about the efficacy of different types of medical care.

Similarly, the recommendation of the competition advocates to modify the tax laws and thereby discourage the trend toward more comprehensive health insurance conflicts with Arrow's analysis that calls attention to the substantial economies of scale resulting from large enrollments in comprehensive schemes and the desirability of removing, insofar as it is possible, the cash nexus from the physician-patient relationship.

No one opposes the reduction and removal of regulations that have come to weigh heavily on the providers of health care, especially when they have largely failed to stem the rise in costs. But modern societies, according to Arrow, resort to political interventions in the health care market not because of their preference for collective action but rather because of their unwillingness to accept the shortcomings of competition. They are determined to find ways of providing access for all to basic health care services.

Arrow also questions the presumed benefits that will accrue from the attempt to force more physicians into prepayment schemes—a major objective of the competition proposals. He presents a twofold caution: the undesirability of confounding the physician's economic interests with his professional role as diagnostician and therapist, and the belief that physicians will take strong evasive actions in their practice arrangements to avoid being placed directly at economic risk.

This juxtaposition of Arrow's 1963 analysis of the limitations of the competitive model and the claims of the procompetition forces of the

1980s should alert those who are looking for the answer to the pressing problem of steeply rising health care costs not to exaggerate the gains likely to result from seeking to make the market more competitive. Competition cannot provide the answer.

STIMULATION OF DEMAND VS. MARKET FAILURE

"The procompetition group" is a misnomer. It consists of a number of academics with little sensitivity to politics loosely aligned with a number of legislators possessed of an unwarranted respect for economics who are convinced that Congress must act to constrain the increases in health care costs, and see competition as the only hope. The common thread that justifies talking of them as a group is that they trace the steep rise in health care costs to "market failure" and that they believe that until the market is permitted to function freely there will be no way to bring runaway costs under control. Each of the reforms that they advocate is directed to overcoming one or another type of market failure.

Their critique of the extant system is founded on the observation that the consumer who purchases health insurance or joins a prepayment plan has little or no incentive to be concerned with its cost. The consumer will choose the richest benefit plan that the employer offers and because of the hidden tax subsidy will, with his union representative, press for ever more comprehensive benefits. The procompetition critics have a point, in fact two points: the tax subsidy provisions encourage the recipients to select the "richest" coverage; and pressure is exerted on current plans to expand coverage to include mental illness, eyeglasses, dental services, and still other "extras."

But this is not the whole story. Tax benefits were introduced to encourage the growth of private insurance. Consumers have repeatedly expressed a strong preference for first dollar coverage in the case of hospitalization, a concept which is admittedly at variance with the logic of insurance but surely legitimate in an economy that honors consumer sovereignty. Furthermore, workers and their leaders who negotiate for them are not oblivious to the tradeoffs between more and better health care benefits and attractive alternative rewards in the form of higher wages, more vacations, increased pensions. One major reason for the steep rise in health care costs has been the continuing preference of employees for more and better health benefits with first dollar hospital coverage.

The pressures on the demand side were greatly increased in 1965 with the public's decision to broaden access to quality health care for the elderly and the poor. Forecasts of the future costs of Medicare and Medicaid proved to be gross underestimates, but that is typical for most public programs—from new weapons systems to the construction of public buildings. The American people made a deliberate decision to spend more on health care through government.

In fact, the entire post-World War II era speaks to the sustained efforts of Americans to broaden and deepen the health care system through large-scale expenditures for hospital construction (Hill-Burton, P.L. 79-725), biomedical research (National Institutes of Health), the expansion of educational opportunities for health professionals (state and federal governments), private health insurance, and public grants, loans, and tax guarantees to encourage accelerated investments in the health care industry.

The American people began a love affair with therapeutic medicine and for several decades asked no questions about the cost of the relationship. Their sole concern was to speed expansion—more hospitals, more research funds, more equipment, more physicians, more support personnel, more financing—more everything.

Leaders in the present administration claim that the preexistent competitive market was destroyed during this period. But it is more consistent with the facts to recognize that health care never conformed to the competitive market. At the end of World War II, the dominant health care institution was the nonprofit acute care hospital with community leaders serving as trustees. Most physicians treated a large number of "no-pay" or "part-pay" patients, and those seeking admitting privileges at teaching hospitals often devoted several half-days a week caring without pay for patients on the wards and in the clinics. Federal and state governments provided a considerable volume of health care without charge to special groups—to those suffering from chronic mental and other long-term illnesses, to veterans and members of the Armed Services and their dependents.

True, physicians and dentists functioned primarily in a fee-for-service environment and the pharmaceutical and medical supply companies were "for-profit" enterprises, but by no stretch of the imagination could it be said that the American health care system of 1950 conformed to the model of the competitive market. In the succeeding decades the gap between the model and reality widened as indicated by the substantial decline in the proportion of health care expenditures paid out-of-pocket by consumers—from around three-quarters to one-third.

The marked departures from the competitive model were deliberate and reflected the expressed preferences of the American people both in the private and public domains. The public wanted first dollar insurance coverage for its hospital expenses; it wanted the elderly and the poor to have access to the system; it believed that large-scale governmental support for research would more quickly find the answers to many dread diseases; it saw merit in providing access to a modern hospital for people

living in small as well as large communities; and it made large investments in broadening and deepening educational and training opportunities to assure an adequate supply of competent health professionals.

In this expansive mood, the public's preoccupation was with increasing
the quantity and quality of health care services and with assuring access
of the entire population to a sophisticated health care system. For a long
time it paid little or no attention to the costs. It agreed to reimburse hospitals on the basis of their costs or charges; and it paid physicians on the
basis of their usual, customary, and reasonable fees, methods of reimbursement that unquestionably contributed to accelerating the rise in
costs. Most of this rise, however, was attributable to the deliberate stimulation of demand. If the competitive market never existed, and it never
did, it is misleading to talk of market failure.

COMPETITION AND COST CONTAINMENT

To what extent are the current procompetition proposals likely to contribute to cost containment for the system as a whole, as distinct from cost
shifting among payers or forcing a reduction in the total quantity and
quality of services available to the American people?

If employees are encouraged to purchase coverage below the maximum
amount that their employer will provide through the monetary incentive
of pocketing the difference, what is to stop the younger, healthier group
from buying the less costly policies, thereby raising the costs for those who
are poorer risks? If this occurs, the total outlays for health care are likely
to increase because of the rebates to the healthier group.

Placing a ceiling on tax free health care benefits will presumably lead to
less comprehensive coverage and this in turn will lead to a lower level of
demand for care because less of it will be prepaid. This may happen, but
several other outcomes cannot be ruled out. Employees may press for
comprehensive plans even if they and their employers have to pay taxes
on coverage above the ceiling. Or they may follow the pattern set by the
elderly and buy supplemental coverage, paying more and getting less for
such coverage than if it had been part of the original package.

If the Gephardt bill (H.R. 850) were enacted and all employees were
given purchase vouchers by their employers with which to shop the
market, marketing costs would far exceed those currently involved in selling group policies. Moreover, many persons in the lower income brackets
might be inclined to buy the least costly policy, assuming that somebody
else—the hospital or government—would pick up the tab if their hospital
expenses exceeded their coverage.

Many proponents of competition are convinced that higher copayments
will moderate the demand for health care services and most of the litera-

ture, including the recent Rand report,[9] suggests that this would in fact be the case. However, such cost containment need not reflect more efficient production and distribution of the current level, but rather a reduction in level of health care services. Such a reduction might or might not be viewed as desirable depending on the answers to the following two questions. Are the American people currently consuming too many, and too expensive, health care services? And would a decline in utilization induced by copayments result in the elimination of marginal services to the overusers or of basic services to justified users? If the latter were the case, it would be difficult to interpret the outcome as cost containment.

The Medicare voucher proposal that has been advanced is also difficult to prejudge. The American Association of Retired Persons sees the proposal as a way to place a ceiling on federal expenditures with indexing for inflation set below the projected rise in health care costs. If the voucher led to a shift in the nature of health care provided the elderly, from high-cost acute hospital care to more home care and community-based services, some cost containment might be achieved.

The procompetition group expects important gains from a reduction and removal of regulations, including certificate of need (CON), which has erected barriers to the rapid construction, expansion, and modernization of hospitals. They argue that CON has been ineffective in controlling capacity at the same time that it has increased costs by prolonging the period from initial planning to final construction. The recent report by the U.S. Congressional Budget Office (1982) confirms that the initial assessments of the efficacy of CON were unduly pessimistic.[10] If the experts are correct in their belief that the country is overbedded, it is difficult to see how freeing hospital construction from all prior assessments of public need would contribute to cost containment. Such a policy would have just the opposite effect of adding to excess capacity, jeopardizing the financial stability of many existing institutions, and resulting in further cost expansion.

The advocates of competition anticipate that the growth of prepaid delivery systems would be stimulated by the foregoing effort to expand competition, which in turn would lead to cost containment. They may be right, but there are reasons for caution. First, the record sheds little or no light on how prepayment plans would serve the elderly and the poor, who together account for around 40 percent of all health care expenditures. Next, the experience of health maintenance organizations (HMOs) in California, Minneapolis-St. Paul, Washington, D.C., and New York City provide, at best, equivocal evidence of their ability to contain costs. Furthermore, one cannot assume that once a large proportion of a community's physicians are organized within prepayment plans, their professional and economic behavior will parallel that of the small number of their colleagues who initially were drawn to prepaid practice plans. But the most telling argument against exaggerated expectations is the probable modest rate of growth of prepayment plans even if the procompetition proposals were enacted into law, a growth likely to be constrained by the preferences of both consumers and physicians for the status quo.

THE MARKET IS CHANGING

The supporters of competition may be grossly overemphasizing the beneficial results that would follow upon congressional action to enlarge the role of competition in health care. But the years ahead will see many significant changes in the health care market even in the absence of legislation affecting competition:

- Federal and state governments will accelerate their efforts to limit their outlays for health care. Governments will probably succeed in reducing the number of poor persons entitled to health care services as well as in cutting back on the services currently provided them.
- As the growth in total health care dollars in the system decelerates partly in response to efforts of governments to contain their outlays, many hospitals will find themselves in increasingly strained circumstances resulting in closures, mergers, affiliations, and conversions. Faced with a leveling off in admissions and utilization, many more strongly positioned hospitals will seek to increase their revenues through diversification: entering into arrangements with satellite institutions, organizing HMOs, and establishing new programs such as "home care" and "hospice care." By the end of this decade or shortly thereafter, the number of unaffiliated hospitals may have been reduced by one-third, possibly more.
- The rapid increase in the number of physicians per 100,000 population, about 30 percent per capita between 1978 and 1990, represents another area of rapid change. When one recalls that physicians receive about one out of every five dollars spent on health care, and hospitals about two out of every five, it becomes obvious that the only way physicians can slow reductions in their earnings in a period of constrained total dollars and increased numbers will be to deflect some of the dollars that otherwise would flow into the coffers of hospitals. Third-party payers will press for more patient treatment in an ambulatory setting. The large increase in the physician supply will facilitate the expansion of new forms of delivery systems which in the past have been hobbled by the disinclination of most physicians to elect an alternative to fee-for-service practice.

- There are few success stories of local health planning aimed at the more efficient use of scarce health resources. In the decade ahead, however, the principal purchasers of health care services, business and labor, are likely to work more closely with the principal payers, insurance and government, to stretch the total health dollar. The large number of business coalitions which are now being established suggests that the decade ahead will be the first real test of area health planning. Although enthusiasm should not be confused with achievement, it would be unduly pessimistic to write this e ort off prematurely.

A decade characterized by constrained dollars, hospitals under pressure, a large expansion in the physician supply, and local health planning is likely to bring about many changes in the manner in which health care is financed, produced, delivered, and consumed. The procompetition forces may be left at the starting gate, but the health care market will nonetheless be significantly transformed. Ours has always been an economy and society more receptive to the forces of reality than the allure of ideas. And we are probably the better because of it.

7

The Grand Illusion of Competition

Greater competition in health care is trendy. Several major bills are in the congressional hopper, and the administration's proposal long delayed may yet be forwarded. The 1982 *Economic Report of the President* referred in passing to "the dilution of competition in the health care industry and the resultant inefficiencies."[1] Economists have taken the lead in developing the rationale for the gains that would accrue from more competition in health care. The *Economic Report* stated that "it is difficult to quantify this loss in efficiency [from the lack of competition] but recent estimates place it in the range of $25 billion a year."[2] To keep this estimate in perspective, it represents 10 percent of total outlays for health care in 1980.

It is important for physicians to appreciate that the procompetition approach is not shared by all economists, probably not even the majority of those who are specialists in health policy. I have dealt with related facets of the competition theme in previous articles in *The New England Journal of Medicine*,[3] *Hospital Practice*,[4] and *Hospitals*[5] (see Chapters 5 and 6), which contain a brief bibliography of economists who have written in favor of or in opposition to competition in health care. It may be useful for an economist who questions the efficacy of the competitive strategy in health care to set out in point-counterpoint fashion the reasons for his skepticism and, in the process, provide physicians and others outside the economics profession with a broader view of the issues under debate.

Competition works reasonably well when a relatively large number of producers, engaged in the output of a standard commodity, seek to gain customers by offering their wares at a lower price. Health care is characterized by the presence of many providers who do not produce a standard

Originally published as "The Grand Illusion of Competition in Health Care," *Journal of the American Medical Association* 249:14 (1857–59), April 8, 1983. Reprinted by permission. Copyright 1983, American Medical Association.

commodity and who do not compete primarily on the basis of price. Just consider the differences in the range and quality of the surgery that is performed in a small county hospital in contrast to the principal teaching hospital of a major medical school. Surgery is surely not a standard commodity.

Competition requires that buyers have access to information about the products being offered for sale and their prices and to have the knowledge with which to judge the relative values of the competing goods or services. Most economists believe that in a specialized arena, e.g., medicine, there is a major asymmetry in the knowledge and judgment of physicians and lay persons, which makes it necessary for the latter to rely on the former for guidance.

In competitive markets, when demand exceeds supply for any length of time, existing or new producers attracted by above-average profits enlarge their output, thereby helping to reestablish an equilibrium. When supply continues to exceed demand, capacity will begin to shrink. In health care, the two principal providers, physicians and hospitals, are not able to respond either in periods of expansion or contraction directly and quickly to such market signals.

The principal regulator of competitive markets is the pursuit of profits, which spurs producers to enter the field and/or to expand output when supply continues to lag behind demand. However, young people who pursue a course of studies that require, on the average, eleven to thirteen years after high school to enter into a medical career cannot respond quickly to changes in prospective earnings. As for hospitals, most of those providing short-term care are in the nonprofit sector, having been organized and built by philanthropy often supplemented by government funds. While they seek to have revenues in excess of expenditures to grow and modernize, they are not driven to maximize their profits.

Price movements up and down are the principal mechanism whereby demand and supply are kept in balance in competitive markets. When prices are increased, consumers restrict their purchases; when prices decline, consumers increase their demand. However, in health care, need is a critical consideration. Patients with symptoms seek medical attention; if they are symptom free, they generally do not seek the services of a physician.

In most competitive markets, the consumer pays out-of-pocket for what he buys, and, in the event that it is a high-ticket item (such as a refrigerator, automobile, or stereo), he may seek credit to help him with the financing. In health care, most consumers have insurance coverage for hospitalization as well as for physician services connected with inpatient treatment to ensure that when they and their dependents need care they will not confront a financial crisis. Since the amount of care they may need is open-ended, most consumers have extensive insurance (for instance, major medical insurance, with coverage of between $100,000 and $1 million). In light of such heavy insurance, prices at the point of purchase have little direct influence on consumers' demand for hospital care.

A competitive market assumes that prospective purchasers are in the best position to know what they need or want and that they will spend their incomes to optimize their satisfactions over the entire range of their outlays. In the case of medical care, the consumer makes only one or, at most, two decisions—the type of insurance policy or policies that he purchases and the selection of his physician. The specific decisions as to the treatments that he will undergo rest primarily with his physician and the other physicians to whom the patient may be referred. The physician acts as an agent for and on behalf of the patient.

Under common law and the antitrust statutes, there are severe constraints on joint action by producers to affect output and prices that threaten to reduce or eliminate competition. While judicial and administrative agencies have recently sought to apply these constraints to the professions, including physicians, the states continue to allow the medical profession wide scope for self-regulation.

In competitive markets, the consumer without purchasing power does without. To obtain goods or services, the purchaser must have dollars to spend or be credit worthy. The government provides income to limited numbers of eligible poor to ensure that they are able to purchase the essentials they need. With respect to health care, our society increasingly recognizes that all who require basic services must be able to secure them irrespective of their ability to pay. The existence of 5 percent to 10 percent of the population who lack hospital insurance and another 10 percent with limited insurance coverage is the size of the gap that remains between the societal goal of access and the ability of the entire population to obtain access.

In the production of goods, competitive markets are usually characterized by constant or decreasing costs, reflecting gains from economies of scale. In the medical care arena, innovation frequently results in life-improving and/or life-lengthening outputs but under conditions of increasing costs. Since the latter represent new outputs, simplistic comparisons between commodity and medical care production with respect to cost-decreasing and cost-increasing behavior are likely to be misleading.

The principal source of purchasing power for consumers in competitive markets is the labor and property income that they have at their disposal. In the case of medical care, the several levels of government account for more than 40 percent of the total outlays, which points to their potential leverage on what is produced and on how it is priced. While nonprofit hospitals have long resorted to cross-subsidization among patients and services to help cover their bad debts, the federal government is increasingly forcing the private sector to cover a greater share of overhead costs allocatable to Medicare and Medicaid patients—the annual cost of which has recently been estimated at about $5 billion.

In competitive markets, entrepreneurs have wide discretion to seek out and use new and different resources to reduce the costs of their output and improve its quality. In health care, entrepreneurs are not free to hire physicians and arrange new patterns of health care delivery, since, under the laws of most states, physicians alone have the right to determine how they will practice.

In markets where commodity trade is preponderant, producers at distant locations, including even overseas producers, often compete with one another. This is definitely not the pattern with health care services. These services are produced and distributed largely in a delineated area by providers that belong to distinctive networks, such as medical centers, large teaching hospitals, small community hospitals, and those that cater to different, segmented clientele—from the carriage trade to the poor.

From the days of Adam Smith down to the new supply side economists, the proponents of competition have stressed the gains that accrue when each producer pursues his own self-interest and each consumer shops to obtain what he wants or needs at the lowest price. However, the medical profession has long sought to restrict and restrain its members from pursuing policies that, while adding to their incomes, might harm their patients. Physicians are under professional and legal pressures to follow "best practice."

Advocates of competition frequently emphasize the importance of restructuring the U.S. health care system so that it will return to the competitive pattern of former days: they are misreading history. Medicine in the United States has not followed the dictates of the competitive market, surely not since the days of the Flexner report.

In exploring the causes of the explosive cost increases after the passage of Medicare and Medicaid in 1965, the proponents of competition emphasize the deviations from the competitive model, since consumers are no longer constrained at point of purchase by out-of-pocket expenditures. However, the procompetition group underestimates the repeatedly demonstrated preference of the American people for first dollar coverage for their health care. Moreover, the group has ascribed too much importance to the absence of copayments and too little to inept reimbursement policies. It has also failed to take fully into account the cost-increasing implications of broadened access to care and therapeutic advances that have also led to cost-raising results.

A major social benefit of competitive markets is the extent to which they are self-regulatory. The government does not need to interfere.

Appalled by the rapid growth of governmental regulation in the health care arena, which has not succeeded in controlling cost increases, the proponents of competition urge the dismantling of most of the regulatory system. Competition should do the regulating. They have failed, however, to demonstrate how intensified competition among insurers, delivery plans, hospitals, and physicians would constrain demand, reduce marketing costs, result in eliminating excessive numbers of physicians and hospital beds, ensure access to the poor and near-poor, and provide funds for innovation. If less regulation and more competition could accomplish the foregoing—and in the process costs were constrained—no sensible person would oppose the reform. However, to date, the advocates have dealt in promises, not in plans and processes that carry much conviction of turning the ideal into the real.

Some of the procompetition group recognize that the fair competition that they seek among health delivery systems requires the government to set the rules about such critical matters as benefits, premiums, enrollment periods, subsidy levels, rebates, and regional cost differentials. If government intervention over such a wide front is a precondition for establishing competition, the question must be raised whether it will ever withdraw. The odds are that in a changing environment, the government will face a continuing challenge to keep adjusting the rules governing competition.

A major spur to the procompetition approach has been steeply rising health care costs that the proponents see rooted in the absence of market discipline and the ineffectiveness of regulation. However, the proponents may be jumping to conclusions. The largest payer, the federal government, is only now beginning to turn down the spigot and prospective reimbursement, and tighter controls over fees are still to come.

The procompetition group argues that health care should be produced under the same competitive conditions as all other economic output. However, they err in failing to realize that such critical goods and services as education, religion, defense, the arts, electric power, and telephone are not produced or sold in competitive markets. The option is not between a health care system in which competition or regulation is preponderant. The real challenge is to acknowledge that our pluralistic system, in which government pays more than 40 percent of the total bill, nonprofit hospitals provide most short-term care, and physicians act as agents for their patients, has many accomplishments that should be respected and protected. True, the acceleration of costs must be moderated, but this should prove feasible through budgetary controls and improved systems for reimbursement. What we do not need is radical reform aimed at establishing competition in health care centered on price rather than on quality. This is not necessary, not desirable, and not even feasible.

PART III

Physicians, Nurses, and Allied Health Personnel

The transition from Part II to Part III is easy, because physicians by law and tradition have long exercised the dominant role in the shaping and operation of the health care system. Their special position and role contradict the theory of the competitive market where consumers exercise the determining voice.

Chapter 8 addresses the question of the probable size of the supply of physicians in the years 1990 and 2000 and assesses the probabilities of action being taken in the near and middle term to slow the potential inflow. The thrust of the latter analysis is to highlight the multiple decision-making levers and the difficulties of developing a political consensus to use one or more of them to reduce the prospective supply.

The long preparatory cycle that must be undergone by students who are planning to become physicians is considered in Chapter 9, which analyzes the views of second-year medical students at one of the nation's leading academic health centers and spotlights the stressful balances they must try to resolve as their idealism comes into conflict with reality.

Even when we acknowledge, as we must, that the 450,000 physicians in active practice in the United States represent the single largest repository of power in the health care system, we do not denigrate or ignore the critical role of nurses, allied health professionals, and technicians, and the large number of supporting staff who together account for about 7 million additional workers in the health care sector. Nurses and allied health personnel together comprise about 5.5 million, or almost twelve times the number of practicing physicians.

As recently as the beginning of World War II, nurses were viewed, and viewed themselves, as extenders of physicians. Their eyes and ears made it possible for physicians to see and do more for their patients. But in the last two generations major transformations have occurred in medicine, in the role of women in the economy, and in nursing education. Chapter 10 explores the impact of economic changes on the future of nursing.

Chapter 11 presents detailed evidence of the discontent which pervades the nursing profession at the present time, discontent centered around pay and career progression, relations to physicians and hospital administrators, work schedules, work stress and even more sources of friction and difficulty. The unequivocal finding that emerges is that unless far-reaching changes are undertaken by all of the parties involved, particularly nurse educators, nurse administrators, physicians, and hospital administrators, the present order of discontent could reach crisis proportions which would place the continued delivery of quality health care at risk.

The concluding chapter in Part III (Chapter 12) provides a broad overview of the large, diversified, and complex grouping known as "allied health personnel," which includes everyone with a doctorate in biochemistry working in a large laboratory to a nurse's aide who has had not more than a few weeks of orientation before being assigned to a hospital floor to assist registered nurses. The physician is currently considered as the only person able to oversee the patient's care and to decide whether, when, and what kinds of diagnostic and therapeutic interventions are indicated. But Chapter 12 demonstrates unequivocally that without the variety of allied health personnel (and nurses), the health care system would grind to a halt. Physicians alone can no longer provide the care that patients require.

8

The Future Supply
of Physicians

Philosophers have warned that a nation that does not know its past will be forced to relive it. We are future-oriented people, disinclined to devote time and energy to understanding the past. However, we would be ill-advised to disregard its lessons.

In the three decades between 1950 and 1980 the physician-to-population ratio in the United States increased from around 140/100,000 to 200/100,000, or by over two-fifths. The best and most recent estimates of the Health Resources Administration, Department of Health and Human Services (January 1982), point to a substantial continuing increase in the remaining two decades of this century, reaching ratios in the high series of 250/100,000 and 290/100,000 in 1990 and 2000, respectively. These numbers translate into a gain of 25 percent during the 1980s and 45 percent between now and century's end.

Reference to these varying estimates indicates that forecasting the future supply of physicians is not a simple exercise. While there is a relatively narrow spread of only 3 percent among the three series (high, basic, low) for 1990, from 242 to 250, the range for the year 2000 is considerably greater, with values of 290, 271, and 266, amounting to an 8 percent difference between high and low.

Attention should be directed to some of the more important variables that confound all estimates of the future supply of physicians per 100,000 population. There is first the question of the size of the population two decades hence. Major uncertainties obscure the future trends in birthrates and the flow of immigrants from abroad. It is much less likely that mortality rates will change significantly.

Originally published as "The Future Supply of Physicians: From Pluralism to Policy," *Health Affairs* 1:4 (6–19), Fall 1982. Reprinted by permission.

In estimating the supply of physicians, one is similarly confronted by uncertain elements, such as the numbers of U.S. and foreign nationals who, after studying abroad, will enter the practice of medicine in the United States; the age at which physicians will retire from practice, partially or completely; the extent to which physicians may at some time in their career decide to shift out of medicine into another field of activity; and reductions in the average hours of work, per week and per year, which affect calculations of the *effective* supply of physicians.

Nevertheless, estimating the future supply of physicians is the easier half of the challenge. the really difficult task is to get some firm ground under the "requirements" for physician services. Some of the critical variables include: the future potential of medical science and the cost of delivering services to the population; the proportion of disposable income and taxes that the American people will be willing to allocate to the purchase of medical care for themselves and for others; major changes in the structure of medical care which may augment or reduce the number of physicians involved in the delivery system, such as a shift from inpatient to ambulatory care settings, and from fee-for-service to prepaid delivery system.

These inherent difficulties in estimating, projecting, and forecasting the future supply of and demand for physicians should be read as a reinforcement of my introductory contention that the study of the past is an essential first step in choosing among alternative pathways to the future. Accordingly, we will proceed as follows. The opening section will present an analytic structure with sufficient detail to reveal the critical measures that the nation took in the post-World War II decades to increase its physician-to-population ratio. It will be followed by a brief examination of the asymmetry between periods of expansion and contraction in the educational training infrastructure that governs the output of physicians. The heart of the analysis will then assess the attitudes and behavior of the major parties that are influential in the formulation of policies affecting the supply of physicians. We will conclude with a consideration of the lessons that may be derived from this exercise for shaping health policy in a pluralistic society such as the United States.

EXPANSION: A RETROSPECTIVE

This section encompasses four major themes: ideas, values, and consensus; money flows; institution building; and human resources. We will assess the forces that contributed to changing each of the four and identify their actions and mutual interaction.

We went into and came out of World War II with a predilection that decision making in the medical arena was largely, if not exclusively, a matter for the medical profession. Roosevelt, in designing the Social Security System in 1935, had conspicuously avoided national health insurance, not wanting to antagonize physicians. Later, when Truman pushed for federal legislation he got nowhere. Although Congress appropriated money for hospital construction (Hill-Burton, 1946) and medical research (National Institutes of Health, from the latter 1940s on), it was prevented by the American Medical Association (AMA) in the early 1950s from making direct grants to the nation's medical schools which were in a dire financial plight. The AMA would yield only this far: it acquiesced to the medical school's use of a portion of their research funds to help finance their increasingly costly educational programs.

It took the better part of a decade and a half and multiple prestigious commissions and committees before Congress acted in direct support of medical education in 1963. The chairmen of these investigations—Magnuson (1952), Bayne-Jones (1958), Bane (1959), and Coggeshall (1965)—with strong support from their committee members, many of them leaders of the medical establishment, labored long and hard for federal action to enlarge the number of graduates from American medical schools.

They were powerfully assisted by growing popular pressure for expansion. Citizens everywhere were encountering difficulties in getting an appointment with a physician, often having to wait for days or weeks. Congressmen, especially those from rural areas, were hearing with increasing frequency from their constituents about the retirement or death of their local practitioner and the inability of the community to attract a replacement.

With Eisenhower in the White House, the AMA was able to restrain Congress from direct support of medical education, but the election of Kennedy in 1960 and the AMA's preoccupation with crushing Medicare finally precipitated a shift in federal policy. Facilitating the shift was the busyness and affluence of most practitioners which finally put to rest their grim memories of the Great Depression, when many young physicians had been forced to work in the post office or to drive taxis in order to eat.

World War II was a major breakpoint in the financing of health care which previously had relied on out-of-pocket expenditures by the consumer, supplemented by philanthropy and government support for public health and chronic diseases such as mental illness and tuberculosis. During and after the war, insurance for hospital care (including physician services to hospitalized patients) took off. The rising real income of the typical family also contributed to higher expenditures for medical care: the public was willing to spend more for the improved therapeutic services that medicine was able to provide.

In addition to substantial annual increases in its research budget, the federal government prior to 1963 made a second contribution to the financing of medical education through large-scale support for upgrading the hospitals of the Veterans Administration which made it possible for them to become affiliated with neighboring medical schools. This arrangement resulted in indirect federal financing for the rapid expansion of residency training.

State governments which, together with selected private universities, had long assumed the principal responsibility for the financing of medical education, were putting more money into the system. This was particularly true in areas that were experiencing rapid gains in population and income, notably California and Texas.

The growth of hospital insurance provided another source of funding for medical education, particularly graduate medical education, that was centered in the nation's proliferating teaching hospitals. The insurers were willing to reimburse hospitals for the costs connected with the explosive growth of residency training, both teaching costs and the costs of paying house staff a reasonable salary. In addition, insurers were beginning to look favorably on reimbursing hospitals for depreciation, thereby facilitating the improvement of capital plant and equipment. These practices became even more important after the passage of Medicare and Medicaid in 1965 since these large new programs adopted liberal reimbursement policies for teaching hospitals.

To complete the account of new funding sources one must also take note of federal and state support in the form of grants and loans for capital projects at academic health centers; scholarships, fellowships, training grants, loan funds, and other forms of assistance for undergraduate and graduate medical education; and the access of large hospitals to the private capital markets to borrow money on preferred items (tax exempt) based on their projected reimbursement and depreciation.

Once the federal treasury was opened explicitly to medical education in 1963, successive legislation provided new funds for capital construction, enrollment expansion, student aid, special support for minorities, start-up money for new schools, distress grants for schools experiencing financial difficulties, capitation, and still other programmatic objectives.

New ideas and new flows of money were prerequisites for changing the institutional infrastructure without which the future supply of physicians could not be significantly enlarged. Because of the long lead time (about a decade) between the planning of a new medical school and the graduation of its first class, it is not surprising that although the number of medical schools rose between 1955 and 1965 from seventy-two to eighty-one, there were only marginal increases in the total number of graduates, from about 7,000 to 7,300. But the next decade, 1965 to 1975, showed far more rapid growth: the number of graduates reached 12,500 in 1975 and approached 18,000 by 1982. The number of schools in the interim has grown to 126.

Thus far we have considered basic undergraduate education. Equally important are the changes in graduate medical education that were centered in major teaching hospitals and their affiliates. Between 1950 and 1980 the number of residents increased from 21,525 (including interns) to 61,819. As has been noted, the hospital reimbursement mechanism that evolved made it more or less "cost free" (surely after 1965) for the individual teaching hospital to start or expand its residency programs and enlarge its complement of residents. Attention should be drawn to the fact that up to the present the nation's residency training capacity has exceeded the output of domestic medical schools. Surplus positions were a strong magnet that attracted foreign medical graduates (FMGs) to our shores for residency training, many with the intention to remain, become citizens, and eventually practice medicine in this country.

In the early 1960s, FMGs accounted for one out of every four residents, a proportion that rose to one out of three in the early 1970s. As a proportion of the total number of newly licensed physicians, FMGs reached a peak of 46 percent in 1972 and continued above 40 percent for several years. In 1980, FMGs (including U.S. citizens trained abroad) accounted for more than 92,000 of a total of some 450,000 physicians, or over one of every five in active practice.

This review of the expansion of graduate medical education and its contribution to enlarging the total pool of physicians provides an easy transition to the fourth theme—the role of human resources. Ideas, money, and institutional growth and adaptation each played an important part in enlarging the supply but we must also note the availability of students, faculty members, and residents to complete the picture. The relatively slow growth of the applicant pool in the 1950s reflected the small size of the college cohort, a result of the low birthrate during the Great Depression. The subsequent expansion was accelerated by an expanded age cohort, a much larger proportion of whom were graduating from college. The final boost came in the 1970s when the medical schools lowered their barriers against the admission of women and minorities. Relatively easy access to scholarships and low interest loan funds reduced to a minimum the numbers of qualified candidates who were prevented from pursuing medicine because of a lack of financial wherewithal.

The multidecade, liberal federal financing of medical research led to a major expansion in the pool of academic physicians needed to instruct the enlarged student body. A growing proportion of the instructional staff was supported on "soft money," but during the long years that such money was flowing rapidly, few administrators and fewer professors gave the matter much thought. The following data indicate the trends in the ratio of undergraduate medical school students to faculty: 1960, 2.7; 1970, 1.5; 1980, 1.3. (It should be noted that most faculty members taught other students as well.)

The principal hospital of the medical school usually found little difficulty in expanding its teaching staff, and even the smaller teaching hospitals that were initiating or elaborating their residency training programs were able to attract competent individuals for positions that combined teaching and practice. The reimbursement mechanism enabled these hospitals to recoup all or most of the generous salaries that they offered in order to secure the talent they needed.

The most striking development on the human resources front was the success of the United States in adding significantly to its pool of licensed physicians following the revision of its immigration statutes in 1965, which made it easy for foreign trained physicians to enter the country for residency training and to remain after they had completed their course of studies.

The complex interaction among the perception that the nation was suffering from a physician shortage, the vastly increased flow of funds into medical education, the ensuing institutional adaptations, and the human resources correlates has been outlined above. What needs to be added are a few observations concerning the indirect and unanticipated changes that occurred along the way. These will influence the period ahead when a policy of contraction may replace the long expansionary era.

The following transformations are not insignificant. Preparation for a career in medicine was transformed from a four-year course of undergraduate study with an additional internship year to an average eight-year course, equally divided between undergraduate and graduate training. The teaching hospital became a major center of educational activity. Third-party reimbursers for hospital care became a principal source of funding for graduate medical education. The new eight-year educational training cycle shifted the center of gravity of the profession from generalists, providers of primary care, to specialists. As a consequence of these major shifts in financing and programming, new power constellations emerged. The most important of these was the academic medical establishment spearheaded by the Association of American Medical Colleges and the specialty societies which assumed control of residency training and specialist certification. Simultaneously, insurance and government became the principal financers of the health care system, together accounting for over two-thirds of total expenditures. The significance of these largely unexpected and unintended results will become evident in the section on behavior where the dynamics of contraction will be described and assessed.

ASYMMETRY BETWEEN EXPANSION AND CONTRACTION

It was not easy, as we have seen, to diffuse the AMA's opposition to direct federal support for medical education, but with that single exception a consensus that the nation should expand its supply of physicians developed with relatively little difficulty. It is unlikely that it will prove as easy to reach a consensus favoring a restriction of future enrollments.

There remain population groups even today that encounter difficulty in securing ready access to a physician, and many patients still complain that their physician fails to give them sufficient time.

Many economists and others who share their views believe that the larger the number of physicians the better, because the cost of a visit will drop and the quality is likely to improve as more providers have to compete for the favor of patients. Further, there is a clear perception among those who seek to develop new delivery systems, particularly health maintenance organizations (HMOs), that a large annual output of new physicians will make it easier for them to recruit and retain graduates who are amenable to salaried practice. If one believes, as most people do, that American medicine gained by reducing the barriers against minorities and women, then a restriction of future enrollments would be counterproductive. On this score alone, many are likely to oppose a policy of contraction.

The principal arguments supporting contraction will be advanced by practitioners with dwindling patient loads and earnings who will look favorably on reducing the number of potential competitors. Some sophisticated payers for health care services, public and private, may also conclude that effective cost control will require constraining the physician supply.

When it comes to dollar flows the picture is equally uncertain. In the past, consumers, employers, labor, and government found it relatively easy to increase their spending, directly and indirectly, for medical education at a time when income, profits, and taxes were advancing briskly. In fact, insurance companies and government assumed responsibility for covering most of the costs of graduate education with no resistance, an outlay that is estimated today at not less than $2 billion annually, possibly more. But it is always difficult to reduce or eliminate expenditures, especially if substitute sources of revenue are not available. So far, cutbacks by the federal government have been compensated in part, if not in whole, by the expanded income from physician practice plans, from increased tuition, and from higher charges to commercial insurance and self-pay patients. But no real alternatives exist if third-party payers decide to decrease substantially their support for graduate medical education.

Consider further the circumstances attending the expansion of the educational sector through the addition of more than fifty new medical schools, the enlargement of others, and the participation of more than 1,300 hospitals in graduate medical training. A medical school with its teaching hospital is a major contributor to income and employment generation. Communities vie with one another to be chosen as the site of a new medical complex and they will fight hard to prevent its loss. Much the same is true for the sponsors of hospitals that were eager to start new training programs once the financial underpinnings were assured. Having made critical changes in their structure and operations, most of them will vigorously resist the reduction or elimination of their residency programs.

Much the same asymmetry characterizes the reactions of key groups—students, faculty, residents—to expansion or contraction. In a society which values free choice of a career for its members, the expansion of the numbers that can be admitted to medical school is viewed as a boon, but reductions will be widely opposed. The additional faculty positions which accompanied the expansion of medical schools broadened the opportunities for a new crop of well-trained researchers to remain in an academic environment, full-time or part-time. While many are supported by soft money, the proportion of faculty holding tenured appointments is high. Although there has always been some alternation between a research and teaching career and clinical practice, members of the basic sciences faculty are usually unable to make such a shift, and if they have tenure, it is difficult to terminate their employment. As noted earlier, patient reimbursement revenues, especially after 1965, enabled teaching hospitals to enlarge their training programs and to provide a reasonable stipend for residents. A cutback in the financing of graduate medical education is certain to create widespread disturbance, particularly among residents who believe that they are undercompensated relative to their heavy share of the hospital's work load and the disproportionate pecuniary gains of the attendings.

More serious troubles can be anticipated if the number of approved residencies were to fall below the total graduating class of domestic medical schools and U.S. nationals who return after undergraduate training abroad. Should such a deficit develop, it would divert and prolong, if not destroy, the career planning and prospects of many graduates, especially those who attended offshore schools.

The purpose of this discussion has been to contrast the relative ease of gaining a consensus for expanding the number of students admitted to medical school in the 1960s and 1970s, with the substantial difficulties likely to attend any serious effort to curtail the teaching establishment in the years ahead. Expansion led to gains for many different parties; contraction is likely to worsen the circumstances of most, if not all of them.

THE BEHAVIOR OF THE KEY PARTIES

We now confront the critical question. Will the numbers completing undergraduate and graduate medical education decline in the years ahead in response to new actions by one or more of the key parties—individuals seeking to enter medical practice, government and other payers who finance most of the costs, or powerful centers in the medical establishment that influence and control the numbers admitted to school and subsequently to practice?

There has been a considerable drop in the number of applicants in recent years reflecting the combined effects of demographic trends, increasing costs, and altered career prospects. The simplest indicator of what has occurred is the fact that less than ten years ago, between 1973 and 1975, medical schools averaged 2.8 applicants for every student whom they admitted. By 1981 the ratio had dropped to 2.1 and there is every likelihood that it will continue to decline consequent to the rising costs of a medical education, reduced grant and loan funds, and less favorable career prospects, both economic and other, when a growing ratio of physicians to population is confronted with constrained allocations for health care.

It would be an error, however, to assume that market signals alone will effect a rapid reduction in the numbers admitted to medical school. At the postwar nadir in 1960–1961 the applicant/acceptance ratio was slightly less than 1.7 to 1. This suggests that, at a minimum, medical schools could sustain a further 20 percent decline in applicants before they were forced to reduce their admissions. The continuing absolute and relative high incomes that physicians earn; the unfavorable career prospects in many competing fields including academia, dentistry, the law, architecture, and government service; the number of upper-middle income parents who can afford the finance a medical education for their children; and the cadre of American students, estimated at over 2,000 per year, who are seeking medical training abroad, suggest that a dearth of qualified candidates is not imminent.

Medical education, both undergraduate and graduate, is expensive and includes outlays far beyond the direct expenditures of students and residents for tuition and living expenses, and income foregone. Therefore it is necessary to assess whether funding that currently supports the system is likely to be reduced or eliminated, and the consequences of such action for the capacity of the training infrastructure.

With the exception of research grants and contracts, state and local governments currently account for the single largest source of support, about 25 percent in 1979, of all outlays for undergraduate education. It is very difficult at the beginning of the 1982–1983 academic year to get a fix on the future actions of state legislatures with respect to their continued support of medical education. Evidence from the recent past provides some clues. A few states have removed from the drawing board plans for new medical schools. Several states that previously bought places out-of-state for qualified students have cut back. A number of states, including

California and Indiana, have mandated modest reductions in admissions. In Michigan and Minnesota, states which are in serious fiscal straits, large-scale plans to modernize their principal academic health centers have been halted mid-stream and are being reappraised. Nevertheless, there is not definitive evidence at this time that state legislatures are considering significant cutbacks in their level of support for medical education. The most that one can observe is that a great many state legislatures, faced with a long-term gap between taxes and expenditures, are looking for opportunities to economize and find outlays for higher education an inviting target. However, medical education, per se, has not yet been singled out for specific retrenchment.

A significant number of medical schools, containing approximately 41 percent of current enrollment, are under the aegis of private universities or are freestanding private institutions. In a number of those institutions with strong research capabilities, federal funds continue to account for a significant proportion of their total revenues. Few parent universities make any sizable financial contribution to the operation of their medical school and in a significant number of cases the flow of funds is reversed with the university capturing some part of the research overhead for general purposes. The critical factors in these private academic health centers are the relationships among the university, the medical school, and its principal teaching hospital. It is the financial health of the last that calls the tune. One generalization can be safely ventured: no private university can tolerate large deficits generated by its teaching hospital.

In a number of states, the legislature provides a considerable subsidy to the medical schools under private auspices. If and when these legislatures find themselves under increasing fiscal pressure they may decide to cut back or even eliminate these subventions which would jeopardize the more vulnerable private institutions.

The role of the federal government in the financing of undergraduate medical education has been declining for many years. At peak, it accounted for 55 percent of the total revenues of medical schools; recent figures point to a much reduced contribution of 29 percent (1979). The financing of medical research has leveled off, in fact, declined, once adjustment is made for inflation; capitation has been eliminated; and grant and loan funds for students have been cut back drastically. There is little or no prospect for a reversal of these trends in the near term.

With private universities in no position to support their medical school and particularly its principal teaching hospital, and with the federal government continuing to lower its level of support across all fronts, the key to the future scale of undergraduate medical enrollments rests with the state legislature. As elected representatives, state legislators will respond primarily to the preferences and pressures of the public and the principal interest groups, forces that we will assess below.

As far as the medical establishment is concerned, one must consider the future behavior of its various components—the faculties of medical schools, the directors of residency training programs, the leadership of the specialty societies, and the active practitioners, a majority of whom are members of the American Medical Association.

It is difficult to imagine circumstances in which the faculties of medical schools would initiate a move to curtail enrollments. In many private schools, tuition now accounts for a significant share of total revenues, about 9 percent in 1979. Reducing enrollments would reduce income and endanger the positions of both tenured and nontenured staff. There may be a few schools whose faculty, if faced with a serious deterioration in the quality of applicants, might move to cut back, but such self-effacing action should not be anticipated.

Directors of residency training, particularly those in large teaching hospitals, will be reluctant to take the lead in contracting, much less eliminating, programs which enhanced their professional prestige, power, and influence locally and nationally. A few may agree with their practitioner colleagues who see the rapidly rising output of specialists as a threat to the economic well-being of the entire specialty and move to reduce the number of residents whom they accept for training. But they are likely to do so only in concert with colleagues who operate training programs in other hospitals and in other regions. Such cooperative action will not be easy either to design or to carry out.

Directors of training, however, will not have the last word. They will have to take into account the actions of a number of groups who today provide much of the funding and support for the elaborate structure of graduate medical education. Through their affiliations with medical schools and teaching hospitals, the facilities of the Veterans Administration fund about 12 percent of the nation's 60,000 residency positions. There are a growing number of indications that federal funding for this large training effort will be reduced, probably radically, in the years ahead.

As we have noted, the major source of funding for graduate medical education derives from reimbursement for inpatient care in hospitals that conduct training programs. Regulatory authorities have made occasional efforts to control these indirect educational expenditures, thus far with little success. However, one cannot assume that past will be prologue. Third-party payers will surely exercise more control in the future over the cost/charge structures of hospitals that they reimburse. They are likely to resist continuing to cover graduate educational costs that exceed, often by a large margin, the house staff required to provide a desirable level of patient care. If they should take such action and if the court and the public are sympathetic, some of the large training centers will have little option but to reduce the number of their residency training slots.

Other forces that may contribute to the reduction of the present scale of residency training are hospital administrators and boards of trustees who conclude that these educational programs have been a major source of rising costs and are no longer required to assure a high level of medical care. Alternative personnel, in the form of salaried physicians and technicians, can be used to replace residents at a lower total outlay.

These potentially powerful financial considerations may lead to reductions in the number of residency positions. But there are several countervailing influences to be noted. Currently there is an approximate balance between the output of U.S. medical schools and the current number of residency training positions. Therefore, any significant reduction in the latter will constitute a major disruption in the system. Further, the pool of 10,000-odd USFMGs adds to the demand for residency positions. Finally, the U.S. medical establishment surely does not wish to terminate the training of sizable, if reduced, numbers of foreign medical students and doctors who intend to return to their native country to practice.

It is too early and the forces operating on graduate medical education too many and too complex to permit a definitive forecast of what lies ahead. A cautious conclusion might be that the tightening of the money spigots is exerting some pressure for contraction but that significant reductions will be effected only if the profession and the public were to reach a consensus that the future output of physicians should be slowed. What is the likelihood that the consensus of the last twenty years favoring expansion will be replaced by a new consensus advocating a constriction of the supply? Such a new consensus, were it to emerge, would require vigorous action by the medical establishment and widespread public support.

Thus far the medical leadership has been disinclined to initiate a call for a reduction in the numbers entering medical training. It has avoided such action as a consequence of the enduring hostility it experienced following its efforts during the Great Depression of the 1930s to limit the supply; its ideological opposition to intrusion by government, particularly the federal government, into critical professional prerogatives; its fear that collaborative action on its part may open it to antitrust suits; and uncertainty whether the prospective numbers of practitioners will really be in excess of market demand.

A few specialty societies in the 1970s addressed the issue of numbers in their respective fields and some took modest steps to limit residency training positions. Recently, the American Society of Internal Medicine (ASIM) has gone public with the statement that a prospective surplus of physicians requires the initiation of measures to reduce the flow of inadequately trained foreign medical graduates into the U.S. health care system. Although the AMA House of Delegates, meeting in June 1982, held an extended discussion on the question of policy concerning the future supply, it decided to reaffirm its existing position.

These signs suggest that the long-term support of the medical leadership for expanding the supply is not eroding. What is more difficult to judge is how long it will be before various county and state medical societies take the offensive and recommend to their state legislatures a cutback in medical school enrollments and possibly even a closure of one or more medical schools, in response to the difficulties of practitioners in maintaining an active schedule and earning a decent livelihood.

One must also anticipate increasing efforts by specialist groups to review the residency training structures in their fields. Historically, residency review has been concerned with considerations of quality, but if specialist groups find that their members are facing a more competitive market with fewer patients and lower earnings, they are likely to shift their focus to future numbers.

The alacrity with which the medical leadership addresses the numbers issue and the aggressiveness with which it seeks to reduce the flow of graduates will depend in large measure on the attitudes and behavior of the public that until now has strongly favored an expansionary policy. In addition, other considerations are that in some states the parents of students encountering difficulties in gaining admission to U.S. medical schools will continue to be a force opposing cutbacks. Similarly, persons concerned about the underrepresentation of minorities in medicine are likely to oppose a shift in policy. A very potent group that will favor the continued high production of physicians are for-profit and nonprofit organizations engaged in the development of new delivery systems to provide medical care. The more graduates, the easier the implementation of new efforts.

But the heart of the matter, as far as the public is concerned, involves two considerations: how a change in the future supply will affect their access to physicians, and the extent to which it perceives the connection between the number of physicians and the costs of medical care. With respect to access, one must postulate that the public will be disinclined to support a reduction in the future supply. Common sense would indicate that if the number of practitioners is reduced, patients will have greater difficulty in getting an appointment or having the physician take the time to perform a thorough examination and discuss the results with them. Given the conventional wisdom which states that the more physicians the lower their average fee, it will require time and effort before the public appreciates the fact that more physicians contribute to higher costs by enlarging the scale and scope of their treatments. It would be unduly pessimistic to conclude that the public cannot be weaned away from its long-term commitment to the virtues of an increased supply of physicians. Nevertheless, a change will, under the best of circumstances, not come easily.

It took the better part of a decade and a half after World War II to develop a national consensus favoring expansion of the supply of physicians. If one dates the initial call for a shift in the direction of constraining the future supply to Secretary Califano's speech before the American Association of Medical Colleges in 1978, a new consensus cannot be expected before the early 1990s. Moreover, we have argued that there is a fundamental asymmetry between the processes of expansion and contraction, and that the latter will encounter greater resistance that the former.

The detailed considerations of the probable actions of the key parties reinforce the conclusion that a new consensus in favor of contraction will come slowly, if it comes at all. The scorecard suggests that it will be a long time before career prospects in medicine deteriorate sufficiently to reduce the number of qualified candidates below current medical school capacity. We found further that medical school faculties and directors of residency training are likely to resist any reduction in the inflow of candidates.

The principal forces that are likely to encourage a change in policy are medical practitioners who will confront increasing competition and lower earnings, and state legislatures and third-party payers that are responsible for the funds required to support the costly educational structure. Their ability to alter the consensus in favor of restriction and reduction in the future supply will depend on an alteration in the deeply held public perception that improved access is contingent upon a larger number of physicians. Moreover the public must become aware of the critical linkage between the number of physicians and the costs of the system. Those who believe that the future supply of physicians will be curtailed, particularly those who expect an early reversal of the long established consensus favoring expansion, have the obligation to specify the changes that they anticipate of each of the key parties. This assessment concludes that an early shift in favor of constricting the future supply of physicians is unlikely, not because such constriction is counterindicated, but because the political and economic muscle to accomplish it is lacking.

9

How Medical Students View the Future

In the spring of 1978 the curriculum committee of the College of Physicians and Surgeons (P & S), Columbia University, under prompting from upperclassmen representatives, agreed to offer a course on medicine and society to the second-year class. I volunteered to teach this course, including two hours weekly of lecture and discussions over a twelve-week cycle. The course was mandatory for all second-year students. The requirements included a written examination based on the readings and a ten-page essay on any aspect of health policy that would reflect the student's views and would not require library research or documentation.

The report that follows is a content analysis of the 150 essays submitted by the students. Dr. Edward Brann, my assistant, and I codified and quantified the responses and opinions of the students on the various issues they chose to discuss. It was expected that the issues raised in the course, as well as issues encountered in previous courses, would influence the students in their choice of topics. The course covered a wide range of policy issues, but focused on health manpower and the economics of health. We did not include the question of medical education or the selection of medical students. The only previous course work reflected in the students' themes comprised a few lectures and readings on the elderly and death.

We can report only what the students wrote, not the totality of their views. Students, like all other persons, when asked or forced to comment, are likely to deal with areas of concern and dissatisfaction. This fact must be kept in mind when reading this report. To illustrate: Seven students wrote in favor of a mandatory program for graduates to serve in slums or rural areas, while only three students were opposed to such a program.

Originally published as "How the Medical Student Views His Profession and Its Future," *Inquiry* 17:3 (195–203), Fall 1980. Edward Brann, M.D., was co-author of the original publication. Reprinted by permission.

This, however, cannot be interpreted as reflecting student opinion, since most students were satisfied with the status quo (no mandatory service) and failed to address this issue.

PROFILE OF THE CLASS

The second-year class at P & S in 1978–79 consisted of 102 men and 48 women. All but five were U.S. citizens. Of the 145 U.S. citizens, 23 belonged to minority groups: nine were black, eight were Hispanic, and six belonged to other groups.

Overwhelmingly, they had pursued undergraduate majors closely aligned to medicine, such as chemistry, biology, biochemistry, premedical courses, life sciences, public health, or nursing. A small group (15) had concentrated in mathematics, engineering, computer sciences, statistics, physics, and psychology; the remainder (21) had majored in the humanities or the social sciences (a few took biology or chemistry as a second major). Slightly fewer than one in four had entered medical school from outside the classic preparatory route. On the basis of our careful reading of the 150 papers, we were struck by the fact that so few of the class, possibly only 10 percent, had spent any extended period (one summer or more) in a medical environment—a hospital laboratory, a health care institution, even a physician's office.

MAJOR THEMES

The most frequently chosen major themes for the papers were: 1) general problems of health care, including the reorganization of the delivery system; 2) the medical education process, including the selection of students; and 3) the future role of the physician and the profession. These three subjects together accounted for slightly more than one-third of the papers. Each of the following five themes was selected by between eight and eleven students: the distribution of specialties, including family practice; disease prevention and health education; health care for the poor; medical manpower; cost containment. The combined total again accounted for just about one-third of the class. Between four and seven students dealt with such themes as heroic interventions and dying; national health insurance; evaluation of health need and health care; health maintenance organizations (HMOs); the elderly; the drug industry. The remainder (about 12 percent) dealt with a wide array of topics including child abuse, laetrile, the Roman Catholic view of contraception, swine flu, and other subjects of contemporary interest and concern.

The foregoing classification of these papers by major theme must not obscure the fact that many students dealt with several issues of current national concern. The following paragraphs discuss the themes identified and discussed by the students, whether or not the topics were their major subjects.

Premedical Education and Selection for Medical School

These were the two most frequently addressed issues; approximately 40 percent of the class discussed one or both. The students' opinions were surprising for their level of concern, particularly since neither was part of the syllabus, and for their almost complete agreement on most aspects of these issues. Only one student of the twenty-four who discussed the competitiveness in both undergraduate and medical school felt that it might be positive or even neutral in advancing the profession. Twenty-three made suggestions for improving the admissions procedure, recommendations that included the desirability of selecting more students from poor families, minority groups, areas of physician shortage, those with more preparation in the liberal arts, those more likely to enter a primary care specialty, those who like to work with people, or those who had taken a year or two off after college. The students universally condemned the competitiveness among premedical students. They claimed that students must sacrifice essential aspects of personality development: "Social maturing and perspective may be . . . lacking." Competition conflicts with compassion and humanitarianism: "When I look around my class and see how many of them I wouldn't want as my doctor . . ." The students thought that many premeds forgot about the world around them and the true essence of learning. Ability to work with test tubes was singled out as poorly correlated with the ability to counsel patients. "I am amazed at the social ineptitude of the majority of my classmates," wrote one student.

The process weeds out the nonconformists and troublemakers and selects the superstudent, "who has never had time to reflect on his or her actions, who knows the rules of the game and plays by them all the way." Or, as another put it, "A warm heart in the absence of top grades almost never gets a person into medical school, whereas the reverse occurs quite frequently." One student argued that premed education left "little room for the reflective, creative individualist"; another suggested that the result is an "intellectually bland student community with little ability to challenge and correct existing faults." Others stated that the acquisition of knowledge was secondary to the pursuit of grades and that many chose subjects considered easy with this goal in view. Other comments were more acerbic, including references to "overinflated egos" and the desire of students to see their peers fail so that they could stand out.

Although many students questioned the severe pressures involved in selection for medical school, even more were disturbed about how the medical education system was affecting them, their peers, and, presumptively, the American public. Such terms as "cold," "calculating," "impersonal," "loss of compassion" were strewn through their brief papers. Several complained about the time constraints, restricted social life, the isolation of the long striver: "It is very difficult to be sympathetic when you have had no sleep for 24 hours."

The following quotes are indicative of their turmoil: "Ethical questions concerning 'the rest' of the society seem counter to the qualities of a good medical professional." "The battered image of today's doctor is a result of what the system has done to the individuals who have had to get through it." Under the forced pace, the "chances for a physician's continued self-awareness and growth become minimal." One suggested that a way out would be to change the curriculum so that the students would have more free time. Some thought that the present system breeds people concerned with fulfilling their own wants, which are frequently in conflict with the needs of their patients. The future physician, one said, is "toughened into a hard, often selfish, professional." Several students noted that medical students are taught to keep the patient ignorant and dependent on the physician.

The intensity of these students' reactions to their experiences is suggested by such statements as "cold professionalism"; "medical school is not exciting"; it is a "long, tiresome chore"; "the backstabbing and competition are incredible in light of the fact [of a] supposedly pass-fail system"; "medical school trains people to keep fighting and learning, not out of a genuine desire to learn, but out of fear.... Everybody is afraid that somebody or everybody knows more, has achieved more, and is better than they are." "Around me, I find a sea of preprogrammed, premed faces for whom relevance is defined as the subject of the next exam, for whom success is equated with numerical achievement alone."

Still others remarked upon the dehumanizing aspects of patient presentations, the death of creativity, the fact that students are trained to function as automatons. The social isolation of medical students is emphasized by the fact that of all the students who complained about overcompetitiveness, each though that he or she alone was aware of the shortcomings of his/her peers. Each critic of the status quo seems to have formed his or her opinion independently, since no writer indicated a knowledge of peers' opinions.

There were numerous references to the financing of medical education, which ranged from the observation that the high costs of tuition contribute to elitism in selection, to the common belief that there is a direct connection between these high costs and the high fees that physicians charge. Concern was expressed about students graduating with an indebtedness of $35,000, a figure that may be doubled for medical students who marry each other. Diverse criticisms were made of government programs, ranging from the constricted nature of NIH support for only the research-oriented, to the inadequacies of the total amount of support that government provides.

On the contentious issue of the medical school as a protagonist of specialization versus primary care, the score was eleven to one against the almost total concentration of tertiary medical care that is characteristic of their training.

Many students thought there were shortcomings in the curriculum and singled out the subjects that were underemphasized or totally neglected. Strong criticism was levied against the failure to deal explicitly with the social factors in health and disease; the need for some consideration of medical economics and financing (a shortcoming that this course was supposed to remedy); the need for more attention to geriatrics and death, and a range of additional issues, including health education, preventive medicine, and patient communication. One student thought that a course designed to foster social and economic awareness could not be incorporated readily into the medical school curriculum: "It is hard enough just trying to stay afloat and maintain some sense of equilibrium without having to concentrate on issues which could have been presented more fruitfully prior to the decision to apply to medical school."

When all of the foregoing comments are considered in perspective, several points emerge with clarity: There is no strong defense of the present system of selection for, and education in, medical school. There was pronounced discontent with the crippling effects of the system on the personalities of the students who ineluctably become obsessed with grades. There was concern that the developmental consequences of the processes and procedures to which they had to adjust would distort their future relationships with patients and bode ill for the future of medicine. Many of the P & S students have serious questions about the system in which they are caught, and a large group thinks that it can and should be improved.

Physician Manpower, Distribution, and Compulsory Service

These related issues, much discussed in the course and in the medical and lay press, attracted comments from twenty-six students. Not a single student mentioned a personal desire to practice, even for a time, in a rural setting or in an urban slum, although two referred to the fact that they were enrolled in the National Health Service Corps. Those who offered reasons for rejecting practice in a rural community or in an urban slum called attention to isolation from medical developments, high crime rates, poor facilities, little social or intellectual stimulation, and an absence of opportunities for career development. One even mentioned his desire to avoid the "God-forsaken rural pockets of America."

Although these students stated their preference to avoid unattractive geographic areas, some felt compelled to offer alternative approaches to meeting these national needs. Their preferred solutions, beyond the few who favored a "mandatory service program," included improved incentives for physicians to work in isolated areas and the expanded training of nurse practitioners and physician assistants.

The students, like the public, accept the fact of serious maldistribution, but they recognize that the solutions will not be easy to fashion and implement.

Health Care as a Right and Equality of Access

Approximately one-quarter of the class addressed the above issue. A minority held health care to be a right: "who has the right to put an arbitrary limit on life-saving technology, even when funds are scarce?" "One group should not have to be chosen over another in the allocation of resources." The six students who expressed this view favored the more active involvement of government in the provision of health care.

A related but more restrained position was advanced by those who thought that the present two-class system is unfair and requires governmental intervention to reduce the inequities. But they did not advocate a national policy of complete equality.

The majority (27 out of 38) of those who wrote on the equity-access theme recognized that these goals are difficult to accomplish, and that government alone cannot assure equality of access or treatment: "The right to health care does not mean a right to luxury service." "It is a naive society that claims to guarantee equal and universal access to health or health care."

Many recognized that before the nation can achieve equity in health care, we must confront the cost issue, as well as assess the need for expenditures for other important social goals such as education or housing. In "no way could our society afford the costs involved in guaranteeing everybody access to all of today's high technology." Since medical care will be scarce, services will always be rationed in one way or another: "With limited resources, improved access for one group can only come at the expense of decreased access for other groups." Whatever else might be said about the basic orientation of these budding physicians, they cannot be charged with being unduly optimistic or strongly reformist about extending a high level of care to the entire population.

The Public's Expectations and Responsibilities
Concerning Health and Health Care

This area of concern was addressed by about one-third of the class. The majority indicated that the patient, not the physician, had the primary responsibility for maintaining his or her health. Twenty-four students wrote that the public expects too much from medicine. Among this group were many who expressed resentment that the public frequently acts with impatience if an instant cure isn't forthcoming. A few noted that physicians are "blamed" for conditions that they cannot ameliorate and that, even as second-year students, they were criticized for not curing the medical ills of society.

Almost three out of every four who dealt with the definition of health noted that it is an error to confuse good health care with good health. Good health goes far beyond the physician's realm of influence. Among those who made this distinction, some wrote that physicians should be trained to recognize the nonmedical factors in health and be educated about their influence. Others advised caution, thinking that such an effort would constitute medical imperialism and extend the domain of medicine beyond the limits of physicians' ability to contribute.

On balance, while the majority recognize that health differs markedly from health care, they opted to stay within the conventional boundaries of preventive, therapeutic, and rehabilitative medicine, looking to other professionals to deal with societal forces.

Physicians, Physician's Incomes, and Related Matters

A significant number of students, roughly 10 percent, addressed the question of what influenced their choice of medicine as a career. The most frequent factor identified was "to do good"; intellectual challenge and fascinating work were not far behind. But of almost equal importance were such considerations as "money" and "prestige," although more students singled out "money" to deny, rather than to affirm, its influence.

Among those who addressed the issue of physicians' incomes, most thought that high earnings are justified by the high costs and attendant sacrifices that students make before being admitted to practice. But a minority questioned the prevailing high earnings, recommending that physicians with high incomes should be forced to justify them; two called attention favorably to the Canadian insurance system, which requires physicians to explain their high incomes to their peers. This has contributed to a recent relative decline of physician earnings.

The AMA was a matter of little or no concern to most of the students; only four dealt with it explicitly at any length, and of these, three were highly critical.

Approximately 10 percent of the class referred to personal experiences as health care workers at home or abroad before entering medical school. Most focused their comments on problems that they had encountered and possible solutions. Two who had been exposed to the health care systems in Latin America and Asia were impressed with their efforts to use limited resources effectively.

Another group of nineteen students cited personal anecdotes to illustrate what they thought about various aspects of the health care system. The most common anecdotes showed physicians in a poor light. Others reported on patients who had been hurt by the system. Two mentioned problems in the operations of HMOs. Others discussed difficulties in the health care system that did not result directly in poor patient care. Only three students referred to an incident that reflected favorably on the health care system.

The only reasonable conclusion from these observations is that the shortcomings of the system were more striking to these students than were its strengths.

Primary Care and Family Practice

Approximately one out of five students addressed this theme, with the majority thinking that primary care should receive more emphasis from all sectors of the medical profession than it does currently. They indicated that the principal gains from more primary care would be more personalized care and greater continuity, both desired and essential. We must add, however, that only one student indicated that he planned to go into primary care.

A significant minority of students stated that family practice and primary care is the wrong route for physicians. "A physician almost has to specialize these days." If more primary care providers are needed, these students wrote, the society should expand the supply of nurse practitioners and physician assistants. "The family practitioner represents a waste of medical education"; "he gets no respect"; "most physicians would soon become bored"; "family practice is an anachronism."

Thinking that more attention should be devoted to primary care, while at the same time refusing to consider seriously entering the field themselves, the majority of these students achieved the following resolution to the dilemma: Medical schools should de-emphasize the model of tertiary care; during admission interviews, more attention should be paid to students likely to be interested in practicing primary care; the profession should consider how the status and incentives of primary care practitioners might be enhanced.

Medical-Lay Antagonisms

Of the forty students who discussed this issue, approximately one-third placed a good deal of the blame for the tension squarely on forces outside of medicine, arguing that the public expectation about the efficacy of medicine is too great, that it's fun to pick on doctors, and that the public expects too much sacrifice from members of the profession. But twice as many students placed at least part of the blame on the profession itself, singling out in particular such negatives as: impersonal care; the large egos of physicians with the glorification of mystique; the failure to communicate with patients; the placing of technology above the art of medicine; and the too numerous "bad apples," including those who engage in fraud.

Government and the Reform of the Health Care System

The majority of students (roughly three to one) who discussed the reform of the health care system favored minor incremental reforms, directed for the most part to specific improvements, rather than drastic reform. This majority thought that on balance the system is doing a fairly good job; one student said that it is "difficult to find a macroscopic effect of the failure of our current system to provide health care to all."

Of the forty-three students who discussed government's involvement in medicine, about one-third noted the need for the greater involvement of elected and administrative officials. Some of their comments follow: "Delivery of care would benefit from some degree of federal control." "There is a national need to single out the medical profession as requiring federal controls." "Government has to see that there is no discrepancy in health care between rich and poor."

Some students saw both pluses and minuses from greater governmental involvement, but the majority were clear that such involvement could have dysfunctional results such as higher costs, bureaucratic inefficiency, and additional red tape. Moreover, some were concerned about government involvement that would "compromise freedom of scientific exploration" and personal medical care.

Quality Control in the Profession

Approximately twice as many students favored internal over external controls, such as mandated review boards, treatment audits, and relicensing exams. Some of those who opposed external controls thought that the main guarantee of quality in medicine is in the selection and training of medical students. They expressed concern that bureaucratic norms and standards might discourage those most devoted to pursuing excellence.

Medical Research

Student views on medical research were most striking by their absence. Even the nineteen students who raised the issue gave it only fleeting mention. As might be expected, most favored an expanded research budget, with the group about evenly split between favoring general expansion and expansion in their own pet areas. Three of the four students who discussed financing of research in some detail suggested that basic research is more important than more add-on technology, such as ambulances equipped to handle cardiac arrests.

Disease Prevention and Health Education

Since these issues have been highlighted in the press recently, it is not surprising that forty-two students chose to address them. Just over one-half gave a rhetorical call for more of each. Of the remainder, more than one-half wanted more research and demonstration projects in these areas. Five students came down squarely against an increased effort, maintaining that those who are concerned about improved disease prevention can obtain the necessary information on their own without an organized (i.e., government-run) campaign, and that those who abuse their bodies are motivated by the pleasures of smoking, drinking, over-eating. One student mentioned that programs devoted to health education are most likely to fail among the poor because life in a poverty setting discourages people from observing proper health habits.

HMOs and NHI

Public attention is, however, no guarantee of student concern. Only thirteen students discussed HMOs, and they were more or less evenly split. Six gave positive reactions to these units, two were mixed, and five had negative views. Only nineteen students gave NHI more than passing mention. Of these, only two supported complete coverage for everybody, and an additional two favored a nationalized health system. Eight students were dead set against any form of NHI because of its inflationary nature, the inefficiency they expect it to foster, and its inability to correct what they view as the basic problems (such as maldistribution) in health care. Seven students favored less than complete coverage, such as catastrophic insurance or expanded coverage for the near-poor.

The Future Practice of Medicine

The sixteen students who reflected on the future of their profession shared a common vision. All saw a greater supply of physicians, less freedom of choice for the doctor and his patient, more government control, more practitioners working for salaries with a concomitant decrease in private practice, and more reviews, paperwork, and bureaucratic control. Only one student viewed the future as rosy.

Most thought that the future will be shaped as a result of a concatenation of errors that occur along the way. They expressed concern that they will be reduced to "compilers of data" and "performers of procedures." Some thought that the dedicated physician would leave the field and promising students no longer would enter it. "Mediocrity will become the rule," wrote one. They expected that the practice of medicine will become just a job, that motivation to achieve excellence will decrease, that medicine will become a business rather than an art or a profession, and that the rewards will not justify the sacrifice. One female student said that she was afraid that her income would be lower than she might like.

Even without an elaborate coding and statistical effort, we found it possible to analyze the differences of opinion among these students along two major axes—by sex and by undergraduate major. Our findings, which are reported in the sections that follow, turned out to be more of a challenge to, than a confirmation of, conventional wisdom.

FEMALE VS. MALE OPINIONS

In general, the papers did not support preconceived views of significant differences between female and male medical students. There is a consensus that women are more concerned about the health of the poor, more interested in so-called soft issues such as health education, and less worried about such matters as government intervention and future personal income. By and large, the women did not differ from the men on these issues. Men were slightly more likely to express their concern over the competitiveness and the inhumanity of their classmates and the system through which they were progressing. Women showed somewhat less concern than men over the extremely specialized nature of their training. Women were more likely to support a mandatory service program and somewhat more supportive of the notion that health care is a basic human right. At the same time, women were as likely as men to complain that the public expects too much from the medical system. Fewer women addressed the issue of physicians' incomes, but all of those who did supported the present level of high earnings. Women were distinctly opposed to external quality controls. They were no more concerned than men about whether additional efforts and monies should be directed to disease prevention and health education.

On two key issues the women did differ from the men. Few women discussed the future of the medical profession, and those who did stated that they expected a much greater degree of government involvement and more drastic reforms of the health care system.

OPINIONS ANALYZED BY UNDERGRADUATE MAJOR

The following paragraphs assess the extent to which students who followed the conventional preparatory course of study (biology, chemistry, or other premed subjects) held different views from those who followed alternate pathways (physics, mathematics, engineering, or the humanities and social sciences). It was expected that those with nontraditional majors would be more interested in social issues and less conservative in their opinions. The results did not bear this out.

The students who had taken nontraditional undergraduate majors were more likely to oppose greater government involvement in medicine. Those who had followed traditional majors were more likely to favor expansion of family practice/primary care. Both groups of students had similar negative reactions to the tertiary-only orientation of their medical school training. Their views as to the future of medicine did not differ. Both groups were concerned about future budgets for research. Both groups expressed equal concern about physician income, and split about equally on whether or not future high personal incomes were justified. Those with nontraditional majors were as likely as the others to put some of the blame for poor health on the patient.

There were some additional issues on which the groups differed. Those who had been humanities majors were far more likely to complain about the competitiveness of medical education, which may have reflected some lesser degree of aptitude for scientific subjects. Those with nontraditional majors were less likely to call for drastic reform of the health system than the other group. Nontraditionals were, however, more likely to suggest that physicians become more involved in politics.

It is likely that those who had followed undergraduate majors in the humanities had more in common with the values and aptitudes of those who followed the traditional or scientific path than with other humanities students. Consequently, the finding that their attitudes toward medicine and society paralleled those of their fellow students in medical school is not surprising.

DISCUSSION

Even if allowance is made for the biases inherent in the selection process, it would be surprising if 150 students in the second year of a leading medical school were to have identical opinions about their education, their occupational choice, their future careers, the larger society about which they still know little, and government, which is a force apart from their direct experience. Still, the differences among them, at least to these readers of their themes, are not large. Let us point out briefly the reasons for our conclusion.

Many verbalized their discontent with the pressures they have encountered and are still caught up in—getting into medical school, the competition in medical school, and the knowledge that they will have to continue to compete for professional opportunities. Almost no one thought that the process was efficient or necessary.

Many noted the gap between the instruction in specialized medicine that is the hallmark of their school and their belief that much of a physician's practice is centered around the provision of primary care. But they have no answer, at least for themselves, about how the gap can be closed. They think that the education they are receiving will be wasted if they turn to general practice, and they expect that general practice soon would prove boring and intellectually deadening. So they remain ambivalent about their medical school curriculum and look to nurse practitioners and physician assistants to provide the primary care which they believe must be provided more widely.

Many pointed out defects, even serious shortcomings, in the current system of health care delivery, but only a small minority advocate major reforms. Most prefer incremental changes.

Many are uneasy about the growing role of government in the control of the health care system, since they think that increasing federal regulations will constrict their freedom to treat their patients as they believe they should. Additionally, they say that government intervention will result in a waste of resources and more bureaucratic infrastructure.

Many think that the public has exaggerated expectations of what medicine can produce and that it has failed to assume responsibility for protecting and maintaining its own health.

After forty-five years of teaching at the main campus of Columbia University, I was surprised at the difference in the academic medical environment, which I encountered only two miles away at the Health Sciences Center. Medical students are indeed a group apart from other students. Despite the superior academic achievement of this carefully selected group, they seemed, at the start of the course, to be surprisingly uninformed (as opposed to ill-informed) about basic issues in the health care field—many could not distinguish Medicaid from Medicare. Their education to this point appeared thin—strong on data gathering and scientific analysis but surprisingly weak in the areas of scientific curiosity and policy relevance. I developed my lectures to encourage them to think about medicine, society, and their future careers. They pressed me for more hard facts and hard analyses. Few students volunteered to participate in the discussions I sought to provoke. They were apparently unaccustomed to this mode of learning. I found them contentious. When I announced that the course requirements would include a two-hour, in-class essay examination based on a broad acquaintance with the required readings, plus a ten-page, issue-oriented essay that would not involve them in library research, I found myself in a confrontation that was carried all the way to the dean.

As the term progressed, however, I came to understand better the system through which students were progressing and the manner in which it shaped and misshaped them. Reading their examination papers and essays led me to a renewed respect for their drive, capacity to assimilate information, critical judgment, and balanced social views. But I could not repress the question of whether their sacrifice of a good part of their youth, their *joie de vivre*, their sleep, and even their friendships and love, for the privilege of studying medicine, would be worthwhile for the majority, given the uncertain future of American medicine.

10

Economics and the Future of Nursing

In a democracy such as ours, every occupational group worth its salt recognizes that, as a precondition for advancing the well-being of its members, it must organize itself. This premise is true for captains of industry, trade unionists, government bureaucrats, and professors, just as it is true for nurses and other health professionals. But it is also true that the success of an occupational group will in large measure depend on the fortunes of both the economy as a whole and the industry to which it is most closely aligned.

Before looking ahead to chart the path of nursing in the 1980s, it will be helpful to cast a backward glance to illuminate the interrelations among nursing, health care, and the economy during the third of a century since the end of World War II. With apologies for excessive condensation, one can identify—among the economy, health care, and nursing, in that order—the following crucial linkages.

After World War II, the United States enjoyed a period of rapid growth, faster than at any earlier period of its history, which resulted in real gains of over 80 percent in income per capita. Since the number of married women entering the work force increased from one in three to one in two during this period, real family income increased even more.

This rise in affluence provided the basis for the spectacular flow of funds into the health care industry via insurance, governmental expenditures, and direct consumer outlays. Annual expenditures rose from around $50 to over $1000 per capita, or more than twenty times. Although inflation has been bad, it clearly accounts for only a small part of this spectacular increase. Rising public affluence coinciding with a period of great progress in therapeutic medicine encouraged the pub ic to seek more and better health care.

Originally published as "The Economics of Health Care and the Future of Nursing," *The Journal of Nursing Administration* 11:3 (28–32), March 1981. Reprinted by permission.

Nusing made significant gains as a result of the expansionary post-World War II environment. For example, salaries and working conditions improved markedly; the relocation of most nurse training into the structure of higher education brought qualitative gains; and the skills and responsibilities of baccalaureate trained nurses were upgraded.

But neither the economy as a whole, nor any industry such as health care can keep expanding indefinitely. Two years after Medicare and Medicaid were passed in 1965, Congress became aware that it had opened the spigot too far, and began to tighten it. With the economy's growth beginning to slow at the same time, the decade of the 1970s has been dominated by a search for "cost containment," although action continues to lag behind words. Economists have lost their brashness. They have learned the hard way that their tools do not permit them to discover ahead of time the success of OPEC, the virulence of inflationary expectations, or the remarkable competitiveness of the Japanese, all of which are among the most potent factors shaping the U.S. and the world economy in 1980. But brash or not, I must set down my best judgment of the shape of the U.S. economy in the years ahead.

In brief, how do I see the years immediately ahead? I perceive relatively slow real growth; continuing high and, if we are lucky, receding inflationary pressures; taxpayer resistance to enlarged governmental expenditures; a slow shift in federal outlays from human resources to defense. It is unlikely that we will confront a more favorable situation. However, it could turn out to be much worse if, for instance, the fragile international money and trade structures begin to give way; hostilities break out in the Middle East; or other major shocks not now foreseen occur.

ECONOMIC EFFECT

What does such a constrained environment imply for the economics of the health care system? There will be no or very little new money (beyond additional dollars required to pace the inflation) available to expand or improve the system. While some fringe politicians and fringe special interest groups are still lobbying for the early institution of national health insurance, there is not the slightest prospect of such legislation in the near term since it would require tens of billions of additional dollars of federal outlays. Such sums are simply not in sight. Considering that NHI first was placed on the nation's agenda by Theodore Roosevelt in the campaign of 1912, some additional years' delay should not be surprising. I have long believed that NHI will be passed if, and only if, the large nonprofit and commercial health insurance system collapses, an event which I do not anticipate.

The constrained economic environment will do more than inhibit funding for expansion and improvement. It will exert increasing pressure on all providers to economize, to cut back, to make do with less—in short, to move from talking about "cost containment" to doing something about it. Since hospitals account for 40 percent, and hospitals and nursing homes combined account for 50 percent, of all health care expenditures, they will be under increased pressure to control and reduce their outlays.

Hospitals and nursing homes are the primary employment setting for nurses, accounting between them for close to four out of every five positions. Since the availability of dollars is the key determinant of how many persons hospitals and nursing homes hire, the outlook is not favorable to increased employment in these sectors and also not favorable to any significant gains in salary and fringe benefits.

Many assume that the United States has too many acute hospital beds—the conventional estimate is a surplus of 100,000. Even a 10 percent reduction of this total capacity would cause a substantial shrinkage in the employment market for nurses. New York City, where the shrinkage of public and community services is not easy to accomplish, has experienced a loss of over 4,000 beds in the last years, a warning that the constriction of hospital facilities is a distinct possibility.

To avoid misunderstandings, let me stress that the foregoing projection of possible shrinking employment opportunities for nurses in institutional settings speaks to economic realities not to the needs or desires of patients for nursing care. My ninety-three-year-old mother was hospitalized twice in the months before her recent death in one of New York's leading hospital centers with a well-deserved reputation for being patient- rather than research-oriented. On both occasions, the hospital's nursing service could not possibly provide her with the attention she needed. We had to arrange for the geriatric attendants who cared for her at home to move into her hospital room and attend her.

Bruce Vladeck, in his penetrating study of nursing homes *Unloving Care* (Basic Books), underscores the crying need for more and better quality personnel, particularly more nurse supervisors. But knowledgeable about the subject, he sees little prospect of attracting them and thus recommends instead elimination of the weakest institutions.

OUTLOOK FOR NURSING

So much for the broad picture. What are the prospects for nursing? While I appreciate that not all nursing leaders would subscribe to the following goals, it seems to me that most are pressing for them.

With respect to the preparation of nurses, the leadership favors a marked increase in the preparation of baccalaureate educated nurses as well as a substantial increase in the number of nurses who complete graduate education to become nurse practitioners.

The second thrust of the leadership is to secure a change in the state nurse practice acts to assure that the expanding pool of nurse practitioners will be able to use their knowledge and skills as fully as possible. On a related front, the leadership is pressing for a change in reimbursement practices so that third-party payers will reimburse nurse practitioners in the same fashion as they now reimburse physicians on a fee-for-service basis. The recent exceptions written into federal legislation, enabling nurse practitioners in federally supported rural and inner-city health centers to be reimbursed on a cost, not charge basis, are a step in the right direction, but only a small step.

The third thrust of the leadership is directed toward assuring that nurses are accepted by physicians as colleagues who can contribute professionally, through a team approach to deciding, implementing, and maintaining a patient's therapeutic regimen. Some of the leaders see an advantage to providing nursing services to hospitals through contractual arrangements between the institution and an agency of their own. Through such arrangements, the hospital will reimburse nursing on a fee-for-service basis, thereby attesting to nurses' role as independent health practitioners.

Let us consider now how the constraints from a slow rate of economic growth and a stringency in funding for the health care industry are likely to impact the three major areas on the nursing leadership's agenda—education, reimbursement, and utilization.

EDUCATION

The education of a larger number of baccalaureate nurses would involve: (1) additional outlays by state governments—the primary source of funding; (2) expanded support from the federal government for the training of additional faculty, scholarship funds, and other infrastructure assistance; and (3) most importantly, the willingness of more potential nursing students (and their families) to assume the substantial short-run costs connected with a four-year program of undergraduate studies.

State governments tend to respond to market signals. If a large number of job openings are available and a large number of young people seek to enter educational programs leading to entrance into these jobs the states are likely to respond. But that does not appear to be the case with collegiate level nursing. Hospitals (by far the dominant employer) are not specifying that they want or need substantially more nurses trained at the baccalaureate level. The number of young people entering and completing nursing programs is leveling off and will decline. The costs of a four-year undergraduate course are mounting rapidly. And the executive branch of the federal government has given repeated evidence that it wants to eliminate, or radically reduce, its funding for nursing education.

Unless most of the foregoing reasonable extrapolations are proved wrong, and it is difficult to imagine why that should happen, the only reasonable conclusion is that the goal of a substantial increase in the number of baccalaureate level nurses is unlikely to be realized in the years ahead.

One caveat: Colleges hungry for students are making a substantial effort to provide opportunities for graduates of associate degree programs and diploma schools to acquire the additional 30 or 60 points to earn a college degree. Two points regarding this development: It is not easy for nurses who are working and who frequently have family responsibilities to find the time (and the money) to accumulate 30 or 60 college credits. More important, many of the colleges that seek additional students do not have a nursing program or one capable of upgrading nurses to the baccalaureate level. Hence, many nurses who return to school to earn their college degree do so without acquiring additional knowledge of skill in their discipline. They often fill up their program with courses in English, sociology, or education—not a serious way to upgrade their professional competence.

OPPORTUNITIES FOR NURSE PRACTITIONERS

The condition of state and federal finance is also a deterrent to the expansion of opportunities for training nurse practitioners. But once again the employment market, more than the financing of higher education, is likely to be the determining factor.

In assessing the prospects for nurse practitioners it is necessary to consider, first, the trends in physician manpower and in physician's assistants because of the partial interchangeability among the three groups in providing first encounter care. The 2,000 completing their training for certificates or master's degrees as nurse practitioners plus the 1,500 who graduate as physician's assistants, equal, in numbers, about 25 percent of the annual output of U.S. medical schools.

However, important changes lie ahead with respect to physician manpower. Conservative estimates suggest that by the end of the 1980s the physician to population ratio will have risen from 175 per 100,000 (at the end of the 1970s) to 240 per 100,000, or by approximately one-third within a single decade. (It took the United States three decades, 1950 to 1980, to go from 140 to 175 per 100,000.)

In the face of slow growth in the total new dollars entering the health care system in the 1980s, the stage is set for a decline, possibly a steep decline, in the average earnings of physicians, something they are not likely to accept passively. One certain response on their part will be to seek to protect their turf, which means that nurse practitioners will find it difficult to expand their practice beyond the groups they presently serve, such as the rural and urban poor—groups among which most physicians prefer not to practice.

In order not to paint the outlook too black, let me note in passing that I expect some new opportunities to develop for nurse practitioners in connection with both industry's greater health consciousness and the inevitable expansion in home and community care for the rising number of feeble aged. But these potential gains are unlikely to outweigh the rising protectionism of the medical profession.

What impact will the impending physician surplus have on the revisions of the nurse practice act and on the present systems of reimbursement? There is little or no prospect that states will rescind nurse practice acts which have broadened the scope of practice to permit nurses to make diagnoses and to treat patients. In fact the dynamics of the situation suggest that with time and good record of performance, the scope for nurse practitioners will be further broadened. However, in states which have not yet acted, the physician lobby, faced with an unfavorable economic outlook, is likely to redouble its efforts to prevent any change in the existing statutes that could affect them adversely.

Although I have no expertise in the legal arena, I want to add one proviso. If there should be a rash of malpractice suits, and if physicians in a supervisory role to nurse practitioners were to find themselves suddenly held liable for large damages, even such freedom as nurse practitioners have been able to wrest may be jeopardized. But on the basis of experience to date, I consider this a minor, not a major, threat.

This brings us to the critical issue of reimbursement and the prospect for change that will enable nurse practitioners to charge on a fee-for-service basis. Federal and state governments are increasingly concerned with gaining more control over their ongoing liabilities for reimbursing both institutions and health professionals. Thus, I see little prospect of nurse practitioners gaining, in a period of constrained funding, what they were unable to achieve when money was flowing freely. The debates surrounding the exceptions Congress made for nurse practitioners in federally funded rural and urban health centers clearly signal that legislators are very alert about the large financial liabilities that would inevitably follow a policy change that resulted in fee-for-service reimbursements to nurse practitioners.

A considerable and growing number of studies have concluded that nurse practitioners do as well and sometimes better than physicians in providing first encounter care; that they tend to elicit a positive response from the patients they serve; and that they are generally cost-effective.

The last point depends very much on the setting the assignments they are given, the nature of the supervision, and still other considerations such as the value attached to such functions as health education, an important goal of many nurse practitioners.

But there is little to be gained from undertaking additional studies to assess these several dimensions of the work of nurse practitioners if the controlling forces of a much-expanded physician supply and a tightening of the financial spigot preclude any substantial redesign in the delivery of health care services which would enlarge the sphere of action open to nurses.

One arena for further investigation might be justified even in the face of the foregoing constraints. The experience of established and new health maintenance organizations (HMOs) regarding whether the use of nurse practitioners is more cost-effective than the use of physicians might yield important insights, especially in a period when physicians are likely to look more favorably on salaried positions.

COLLEGIALITY

We now confront the third goal which, in oversimplified form, can be viewed as a fundamental change in the attitude and behavior of physicians, hospital administrators, and others in authority toward nurses. Instead of treating nurses as underlings whose eyes and hands they command, physicians are being pressed to consider them as colleagues and to grant them a role in collegial decision making affecting the welfare of patients.

As an outsider listening with a third ear, this is what I hear: Nurses have engaged in a struggle for professional emancipation for many decades, but their progress has been slow because of the difficulties they have experienced in defining their area of expertise, in adding significantly to it through research and development, in differentiating who among the 2.5 million individuals engaged in nursing and nursing support services are to be treated as professionals, and in resolving many more unanswered and probably unanswerable questions.

But many of the continuing difficulties lie not with nurses but with physicians. Persons at the top of the totem pole often come to assume that they are there by virtue of right, not as a result of history and tradition. They are loath to cede any part of their authority and privilege and they see no reason why what was should not continue to be. Medicine has long been characterized by a machismo ethic, a milieu within which physicians fail to recognize that a revolution has occurred in the role of women, particularly the role of educated women, in society and the economy.

There appears to be a growing hostility, dissatisfaction, and alienation among nurses with collegiate and higher degrees—and many with lesser credentials—regarding their on-the-job relations with physicians and hospital administrators. One prophecy can be ventured. The idealized conditions of a former era to which so many physicians hark back will definitely not return.

CONCLUSION

One final word: the advancement of challenging goals is never easy, even when the money spigots are open. The fact that they are likely to be further tightened, if not closed, in the years ahead, will add to the difficulties that nursing faces. But there is still considerable room for maneuver in a health care system which will spend about $400 billion in 1984 and where nursing personnel represent almost one out of every three persons in the health care arena. The challenge to the leadership is to reassess its agenda in the face of these straitened circumstances and to explore which goals can best be pursued and achieved in such an environment. Adversity need not be an impassable obstacle to progress.

11

Nurse Discontent

Searching for realistic solutions to the problems of nurse discontent and nursing shortages requires that we evaluate available data in light of situations and trends affecting the profession. Using this approach, we assess the pitfalls of some current approaches to problem resolution and propose two alternatives which we believe hold more promise for increasing nurse retention.

THE JACKSONVILLE SURVEY FINDINGS

In 1980, the Conservation of Human Resources, Columbia University, in collaboration with the Office of Nursing Education, Jacksonville Health Education Programs, initiated a survey of the nurse population in the five-county area surrounding Jacksonville, Florida. A questionnaire, aimed at eliciting objective and attitudinal data concerning graduate nurses' satisfactions and dissatisfactions with their jobs and careers, was mailed to 6,277 registered nurses listed as licensees by the State Board of Nursing.

Of a total of 1,921 respondents, 1,420 (74 percent) were working as nurses, and an additional 337 (18 percent) were not employed in nursing but, nevertheless, maintained an active license. When compared to other surveys, our findings revealed no surprises in terms of such demographic data as sex, race, marital status, and age.

Originally published as "Nurse Discontent: The Search for Realistic Solutions," *The Journal of Nursing Administration* 12:11 (7–11), November 1982. JoAnn Patray, Ph.D., Miriam Ostow, and Edward Brann, M.D., were co-authors. Reprinted by permission.

Nurses Employed in Nursing

Hospitals were cited as the major work setting for 72 percent of those respondents who were employed as nurses; most perform front-line duty either as staff nurses (50 percent), or general duty nurses (6 percent). About three out of four work full time, all year. Over half of those presently employed in nursing have been in the field for ten years or longer, though not necessarily continuously. And, very few plan to withdraw from nursing in the near future.

Of those nurses employed full time, all year, about three out of five earn between $10,000 and $15,000 annually. The largest number of high earners work in hospitals; however, the settings with the greatest proportion of high earners are nursing education and business/industry (see Table 11.1). These settings also show the strongest correlation between years in the field and higher salaries. Relating education to both position level and earnings among our respondents, we concluded that more education leads to higher positions, and education pays off with increased earning power, but not spectacularly.

Direct patient care was reported as the primary task, in terms of time, by only 55 percent of the respondents. About one in five indicated they

Table 11.1   Annual Earnings from Nursing by Current Work Setting
(includes part-time nurses)

Work setting/agency	Less than 5,000		5,000– 9,999		10,000– 14,999		15,000– 17,999		18,000– 24,999		25,000 +		Total	
	No.	%	No.	%	No.	%	No.	%	No.	%	No.	%	No.	%
Hospital	64	6	148	15	511	51	163	16	104	10	13	1	1,003	100
Nursing home	9	11	25	32	32	41	13	16	0	0	0	0	79	100
School/college health	1	4	9	39	7	30	1	4	4	17	1	4	23	100
Home health agency	4	10	5	12	23	55	9	21	1	2	0	0	42	100
Outpatient clinic	6	8	9	13	38	53	11	15	6	8	2	3	72	100
Nursing education	0	0	3	8	6	16	14	37	8	21	7	18	38	100
Doctor's office	23	20	31	27	54	47	4	3	3	3	1	1	116	100
Private duty	5	17	15	50	6	20	2	7	2	7	0	0	30	100
Business/industry	11	15	5	7	24	32	19	26	14	19	1	1	74	100
Health department	1	2	8	13	42	67	6	10	6	10	0	0	63	100
Total	124	8	258	17	743	48	242	16	148	10	25	2	1,540	100

Percents may not add to 100 due to rounding.

would prefer to spend more time at other tasks including direct patient care (44 percent), and patient education and counseling (47 percent).

One-third of the respondents reported substantial dissatisfaction with their job, and an even higher proportion, about one-half, held a negative view of nursing as a career. Only one in five expressed strong satisfaction with both job and career.

Of great significance to the future of nursing is the fact that 49 percent of all respondents said that they would not choose nursing if they were starting a career now; and 44 percent would not advise a young person to study nursing.

A number of the survey questions addressed the causes of dissatisfaction with work and career, and the replies revealed that lack of money is the number one concern. More money is also the preferred remedy. Also, in an open-ended listing of reasons for negative feelings about nursing, three out of four respondents listed salary concerns.

Money was not the only source of difficulty cited. Ranked second was recognition for the quality of care provided. Hours and scheduling ranked third. The fourth area of dissatisfaction reflected a combination of the first and second—too much responsibility with too little monetary return. Stress was the fifth most frequently cited factor.

Nurses not Working in Nursing

About two-thirds of the respondents not currently working in the field maintain an active license. Over one-third are otherwise employed, the majority full time. Most of those not professionally employed are still in their prime working years. And, it would be wrong to think of these non-working RNs as having withdrawn permanently from professional life since half of them (242) expect to reenter nursing in the near future.

Far and away the most important reason given for interrupting a nursing career was family responsibilities, followed by dissatisfaction with hours and pay which was considered inadequate for the effort required.

ANALYSIS AND COMPARISON

With respect to labor market behavior, there is little difference between the nurses in Jacksonville and elsewhere. While most nurses will stay in nursing at least for a period of years, many will change jobs at fairly frequent intervals, moving among hospitals and between the hospital and other sectors. Such frequent job mobility reflects not only nurses' dissatisfaction with their current employment, but also the low value attached to seniority and the ready availability of alternative jobs. This heavy turnover carries a substantial cost to the employer in terms of reduced productivity until newly hired nurses adapt to the new institution.

Most nurses when they work, work full time, all year, although the fact that nationally as many as one-third work part time is in striking contrast to other professions where most members work full time on a year-round basis.

In assessing the future of their profession, the North Florida nurses appear fairly conservative (see Table 11.2). Half or more of the respondents were strongly opposed to three policy positions that are frequently advanced: greater delegation of bedside nursing tasks to LPNs and nursing assistants; required baccalaureate training for entry into the profession; and providing nursing services to hospitals through outside agencies rather than as employees. Only one proposal elicited strong approval—more organizational activity to further professional enhancement—the emphasis being on organizational, not union activity.

Jacksonville nurses convey the impression that they are more satisfied with their primary assignment of providing bedside care and less con-

Table 11.2   Responses to Policy Statements (in percent)

	Strong Agreement	Moderate Agreement	Moderate Disagreement	Strong Disagreement
Most bedside nursing should be performed by LPNs and nursing assistants under supervision.	18	18	21	44
All RNs should have a BS degree.	20	14	15	52
More nurses should be trained as nurse practitioners.	27	30	22	21
Nurse practitioners should be reimbursed in the same way as MDs.	35	27	18	20
Nurses should provide services to hospitals through agencies, not as employees.	9	12	19	60
Nurses should engage more in organizational activities to improve status, salary, and working conditions.	59	22	8	11

cerned than nurses in other parts of the country with restructuring nursing education to correspond with varying nursing practice levels.

Low earnings lie at the heart of the widespread dissatisfaction which the nurses in our survey expressed with their jobs and with nursing as a profession. They considered that their low earnings were particularly unfair because of the importance and the quality of the care that they provided. They also experienced dissatisfaction with their hours and scheduling, the more so because of stresses on the job.

An extreme degree of salary compression, with small rewards for increased education and seniority, are the hallmarks of the profession. Data from the 1977 National Survey of Nurses support the conclusion that concerns about salary figure heavily in nurses' temporary or permanent withdrawal from the profession.[1] An interesting finding in the Jacksonville survey was that employed and not employed nurses reported very similar total family earnings, $23,402 versus $21,910, respectively. Those who were not working had spouses with higher earnings.

But if we narrow the focus of concern to the questions of whether nurses are reasonably satisfied with their work and career, and if not, what are the principal sources of their dissatisfaction, we find a marked parallel between the Jacksonville nurses and those in other areas. Discontent among nurses runs high. The cause is clear—insufficient money, compounded by difficult hours and scheduling and too little recognition. Wandelt's attitudinal study of 3,500 Texas nurses found salary ranked number one among their dissatisfactions. "Highly ranked" but not in the top ten were family responsibilities, undesirable work schedules, an environment that does not provide a sense of worth as a member of the health care team, lack of positive professional interaction with physicians, and the underemphasis of individual patient care.[2] Weisman's study of hospital nurse turnover in Baltimore found that degree of "perceived autonomy" was the best indicator of a nurse's satisfaction and the best clue to his or her leaving. Respondents in Weisman's survey did not stress current salary per se (many were new graduates working in university hospitals to gain experience) but expressed strong dissatisfaction with hours, scheduling, opportunities for advancement, and prospects for future earnings.[3]

The dropout rate from the nursing profession is much higher than most of us recognize. The 1977 National Survey found that about 70 percent of all licensed RNs are currently employed in nursing. However, that figure is misleading on two fronts. First, many inactive nurses who do not plan to return to nursing permit their license to lapse. The 1970 census found that the number of individuals designating themselves as nurses exceeded the total of current licensees by 20 percent.[4] Consequently the overall labor-force participation rate for the profession might be as low as 56 percent (70 percent of the 80 percent who are still licensed). But even this 56 percent participation rate could be misleading because a high proportion of those employed are probably recent graduates. The dropout rate for older nurses must be very high, which suggests that the nursing shortage will worsen in the future as a result of likely decrease of nursing school enrollments, which will produce fewer graduates, and the higher rates of withdrawal among recent graduates over time.

CONCLUSIONS

Our concluding observations, which follow, result not only from the Jacksonville survey and related studies, but also from my ongoing concern with the problems of nursing since World War II.[5] The following comments also draw heavily on the Conservation of Human Resources' continuing studies of the changing characteristics of U.S. labor markets and, in particular, the development and utilization of health personnel.

The third quarter of this century has seen major changes in the parameters affecting nursing:

- Vast expansion of the health care system in terms of volume, intensity, dollars, and personnel.
- The proliferation of all types of nursing personnel from aides to LPNs to RNs with advanced degrees.
- Changes in women's behavior in the labor market, marked by striking increases in employment rates among married women and the advance of women into many professional fields from which they had previously been excluded or accepted only in token numbers.
- Active support by many nursing leaders for raising educational preparation requirements and increasing professional independence from physicians.

In the coming decade, any attempt to eliminate the widespread discontent that nurses currently express will confront an environment having the following characteristics:

- Severe and continuing pressures for health care cost containment.
- A marked increase in the ratio of physicians to total population that will reinforce physicians' historic opposition to nurse ' aspirations to work as independent practitioners. (The lower end of the physician income spectrum will be closer to the upper end of the nursing range than it has been for decades.)
- An absolute decline of about one-sixth in the number of young people of college entrance age.
- Increased opposition to immigration of foreign workers.
- Further advancement of women into high paying occupations and professions.

• The necessity in many families for two wage earners to achieve or maintain a desirable standard of living.

Reducing or eliminating nurses' growing discontent with their pay, working conditions, and career opportunities will not be easy during the next ten years, when health dollars will be scarce, physicians will be under increasing competitive pressure as their numbers expand, and college-educated women will confront expanding career opportunities. Some of the proposed solutions to the nursing shortage and nurse dissatisfaction will meet with little success as they encounter these constraints. Scant relief can be expected from the following strategies:

Intensified recruitment into nursing schools. Nursing schools already encounter difficulty attracting adequately prepared candidates. In the face of a substantial shrinkage in the age group preparing for work and the broadening of career opportunities for able women, the problem will increase.

Higher credentialling requirements. The baccalaureate degree requirement for RN licensure can only exacerbate the shortage given the softening recruitment outlook that lies ahead. This proposal has already met with limited support under more favorable external conditions.

Redistribution of responsibility and rewards. Satisfying hospital nurses' demands for higher salaries and for expanded roles in institutional policy making will be especially difficult as hospitals and physicians face increasing competition and lower revenues and earnings.

Greater reliance on unskilled personnel. Hospital administrators' intensified efforts to meet their nursing needs by hiring untrained or partially trained persons and providing them with basic nursing skills through on-the-job training cannot provide the range and depth of nursing skills that a hospital requires given the growing sophistication of health care.

Substantial overall salary increases. This preferred solution of rank and file nurses faces hard sledding in a period of cost containment. Hospital nurses salaries alone now account for about $35 billion annually and influence substantially another $35 billion in hospital personnel costs.

RECOMMENDATIONS

If none of these five proposed remedies is likely to prove successful, what are the alternatives? Two approaches appear most promising.

First, hospital administrators, the medical staff, and the nursing staff must conjointly restructure nursing services to assure that assignments and responsibilities are graded to experience and competence. Salary differentials must be appropriate and meaningful, so that a nurse with fifteen to twenty years of experience who has demonstrated competence and motivation can earn at least twice the salary of a new graduate.

More particularly, promotion and increased earning power should be facilitated within the staff nurse job category, so that higher earnings and prestige are not limited to educational and administrative positions. With greater rewards for seniority, nurses will be less likely to withdraw from nursing because they are "going nowhere." Moreover, they may suffer financially by shifting out of nursing. The few existing career level pro-grams, such as the "levels of practice" program, at Rush-Presbyterian-St. Luke's Medical Center in Chicago, seem to stop considerably short of these goals, since salary differentials are small, and every nurse would probably advance to the top level in a relatively short period of time.[6]

Second, hospital administrators and physicians can respond affirmatively to nurses' legitimate desires for broader participation in clini-cal decision making. There is considerable room for nurses to assume greater responsibility both in hospital administration and in the manage-ment of individual patients at the nursing unit level without threatening hospital administrators or physicians. While increased participation, by itself, will not significantly reduce current discontent, failure to respond meaningfully may thwart other positive actions.

Some additional efforts are likely to reinforce these two major approaches:

- Hospitals must make provisions for the continuing education of career nurses so that all who are able and interested have opportuni-ties for upgrading their professional skills and knowledge.
- Hospitals and nurses must seek ways, such as appropriate rotational policies, to prevent "burnout" of nurses with special skills.
- Chief nursing executives should be encouraged to experiment with innovative scheduling, salary arrangements, and the use of supple-mental staffing agencies to obtain adequate coverage for unpopular shifts. The existing and prospective supply of nurses hould suffice if a broad range of work schedules is available. Many hospitals, such as the St. Joseph Medical Center in Burbank, California, have reported great success by meeting nurses' scheduling and salary preference.[7]

Through reduced turnover and improved retention of competent nurses, institutions should recapture some part of the additional cost involved in implementing the foregoing recommendations.

No one can guarantee that if these approaches are followed—career ladders with widened salary differentials, a greater role for nurses in clini-cal decision making, opportunities for continuing education and upgrad-ing, improved patterns of nurse deployment and innovative work schedul-ing assignments—nursing supply problems and widespread discontent will be resolved. But, it is a fair guess that in a constrained environment this agenda for reform has much to offer.

12

Allied Health Personnel

At the turn of the twentieth century physicians accounted for about one out of every three health workers. At the beginning of the 1980s the comparable ratio is approximately one out of sixteen. If one considers all health workers except the physician (and the dentist) as "allied" then clearly the expansion of allied health personnel (AHP) has played a critical role in the evolution of twentieth-century medical care in the United States.

It is not customary, however, to include within the category AHP the following health practitioners: optometrists, pharmacists, podiatrists, veterinarians, and registered nurses. Less agreement exists whether to include licensed practical nurses and nurses aides, emergency medical technicians, and other health and health-related professionals and technicians including persons employed in environmental control, midwives, nutritionists, and medical secretaries.

The answer depends on whether the health care industry is defined broadly or narrowly and secondly whether all persons within the industry irrespective of their occupational designations are included or whether only individuals in health care occupations are counted. To illustrate: Is an accountant employed in a hospital to be included and a nurse employed by an insurance company excluded?

The principal reason for raising these classification issues is to emphasize the wide range of estimates about the total number of persons employed in health care—from a low of around 5.5 million to a high of close to 8.0 million and a correspondingly wide range in the numbers classified as AHP.

This chapter is an abridged form of "Allied Health Resources," in David Mechanic, ed., *Handbook of Health, Health Care, and the Health Professions* (New York: The Free Press, 1983), pp. 479–494. Copyright 1983, The Free Press, a division of Macmillan, Inc. Reprinted by permission.

This chapter follows the conventions and the data presented in *A Report on Allied Health Personnel,* hereafter HEW Report.[1] The HEW Report estimates the number of health workers employed in the United States in 1978 at 5.4 million was distributed as follows:

Health practitioners	1.8
Allied health personnel	1.0
Other health personnel	2.6

Over 60 percent of the last category consists of licensed practical nurses (500,000) and nursing aides and orderlies (1,100,000). Another sizable group consists of 270,000 emergency medical technicians. If these three groups are included within allied health the new subtotal comes to just under 3 million, or approximately three out of every five health workers, which is a reasonable measure of AHP in the United States at the beginning of the 1980s.

Table 12.1, adapted from the HEW Report, sets out the principal categories of AHP about which there is no dispute.

STRUCTURE AND FUNCTIONS

The single largest group of AHP consists of laboratory workers, a reflection of the transformation of U.S. medicine from handholding to active intervention, based on advances in knowledge and technology, resulting in the heavy use of the laboratory for diagnosis and therapy. An additional factor speeding the expansion of laboratory personnel has been the growing importance of the hospital, which facilitated both heavy concentration of sophisticated equipment and the employment of persons with modest education and training able to carry out under supervision a wide array of standardized procedures. Since laboratory tests for inpatients are generally paid for in full by third parties, barriers to widespread use of tests have been largely removed.

Similar considerations, with some modification, help to explain the more than 100,000 radiologic workers. Here too technology has been in the driver's seat, a technology used not only for diagnosis but also for therapy both within the hospital setting and in physicians' offices. Physicians early discovered that they could train assistants who could prepare patients for radiologic examination as well as operate the machines. Radiologists recognized that their gross and net incomes could be substantially enlarged by their employing one or more trained assistants to perform these routine tasks so that they themselves could devote more time to reading the plates and determining appropriate therapeutic interventions for their patients.

Table 12.1   Allied Health Personnel: Key Groups

Laboratory workers, total	240,000	
Medical technologists		125,000
Cytotechnologists		7,000
Medical laboratory technicians		12,000
Other laboratory workers		96,000
Dental auxiliaries, total	231,000	
Hygienists		35,000
Assistants		149,000
Laboratory technicians		47,000
Radiologic service workers	104,000	
Medical records, total	80,000	
Administrators		12,000
Technicians		68,000
Respiratory therapy workers		52,000
Speech pathology-audiologists		36,000
Dieticians		28,000
Technicians		4,000
Physical therapists		30,000
Occupational therapists		15,000
Physicians assistants (primary care)		6,000
Other Allied Health including assistants in optometry, orthopedics, podiatry, pharmacy, rehabilitation, etc.		200,000

Developments in instrumentation requiring close and continuing monitoring of intricate respiratory machines explains the large number of workers in respiratory therapy, one of the newer breakthroughs in contemporary medicine. Earlier, patients who had been placed in an oxygen tent or fitted with an oxygen mask required only periodic observation; the more advanced respiratory equipment requires full-time personnel capable of immediate responses to signals from the control mechanisms. Once again, advances in technology have made it possible for therapists to delegate responsibility for many of these procedures to assistants.

The large number of dental auxiliaries, about two for each dentist, reflects the widespread recognition on the part of the dental profession in the post-World War II era that dentists could substantially increase their productivity and earnings by using helpers. Moreover, dentists could also increase their work satisfaction by passing down to their assistants the cleaning of teeth and other routine activities. The almost 50,000 laboratory technicians represent a related, but distinguishable specialization, once removed from direct patient treatment. Dental laboratories were established and technical personnel trained and employed to prepare dentures, crowns, and other special inlays at a volume that permits economies of scale, with one laboratory supporting a considerable number of dentists who practice within the same or adjacent areas.

How does one explain the different ratios of dental auxiliaries to dentists (2:1) and physicians assistants to primary-care physicians (1:9)? Several points suggest themselves: technical procedures play a larger role in the practice of dentistry than in medicine since in the latter history-taking and diagnosis are critical aspects of patient-physician interchange. The aforementioned ratios also hide the fact that physicians make use of large numbers of helpers in their office practice, roughly two for every physician and more if laboratory personnel involved in serving ambulatory patients are taken into account. Broad-scale consumer acceptance of physicians assistants remains an open question while there is little or no reported resistance to the use of dental auxiliaries, at least not up to the point of their engaging in expanded functions.

The fact that during the course of a year approximately 39 million persons are admitted to a hospital (37 million to a short-term hospital) and that over $140 billion annually is expended on their care helps to explain the sizable number of AHP engaged in record keeping, either as administrators or staff. Since records are critical for physicians' decisions, reimbursement, quality control, and evidence in the event of malpractice suits, small wonder that the record-keeping function requires so many technicians and supervisors.

The concentration of large numbers of patients in hospitals, many of whom require special diets explains the sizable number of dieticians and dietetic technicians. While the total number looks sizable, it averages out to more than one dietician for 250 patients, a modest figure when one realizes the proportion of patients who have special needs and the further fact that dieticians frequently oversee the entire food service for patients and employees alike.

Physical and occupational therapists together with speech pathologists and audiologists represent a manpower response to the development of specialized therapeutics beyond the province of the medical practitioner but inside of modern medicine. These therapies required a considerable degree of technical skill but do not require the practitioner to be well versed, as physicians are, in the biomedical sciences. These therapists have considerable scope for independent judgment even though they depend on physicians to refer patients and to prescribe the type of treatment patients are to receive. While many of these practitioners are employed by institutions, particularly hospitals, many others treat mostly ambulatory patients in an office setting.

The large catch-all category, amounting to about one in five AHP, reflects the wide range of assistants who are closely linked to health practitioners in the fields of optometry, podiatry, pharmacy, and veterinary medicine as well as in certain specialized branches of medicine including pediatrics, orthopedics, rehabilitation and still others.

RECRUITMENT, EDUCATION, AND TRAINING

Up to the mid-1960s employers, in the first instance, hospitals and, secondarily, physicians and dentists, were the primary trainers of AHP. Hospitals had no alternative to undertaking the training of the increasing numbers of technicians to back up and assist physicians in the laboratory, in the X-ray department, and in operation of new equipment used to monitor seriously ill patients concentrated in intensive-care units. Most of these training programs were initially not accredited; the faculty consisted of knowledgeable hospital staff who were persuaded to take on the additional duty of instruction; the numbers trained, except in large institutions, were quite small since each hospital sought only to meet its own requirements; most trainees were employees who were already on the payroll.

But this long-established training pattern was radically altered in the sixties, which saw the proliferation of junior and community colleges whose primary claim for public financing was to provide students with a "salable" skill. The infusion of new money into the provision of health care services precipitated a greatly increased demand for health workers which provided the community college movement with the incentive it needed to move into the breach. And breach it was, because many hospitals were not in a position to expand their training and many smaller institutions were disinclined to start.

Economics played a role. Many hospitals that had long sponsored diploma schools of nursing discovered that the operation was costly and that they stood to gain if nurse training was moved into the postsecondary educational structure. The same thinking applied to AHP. Further, some of the educational leaders of AHP, convinced that the quality of student preparation could be significantly improved if training were centered in university health science centers, urged their states and the federal government to support this move. They argued that the university would provide an environment conducive to the development of core curricula and broad faculty competence in the training not only of AHP but also of all health professionals.

The expansion of AHP at both junior and senior colleges appeared attractive for another reason. More and more young Americans were desirous of obtaining college degrees while at the same time strengthening their preparation for the labor market. The movement of education for AHP out of the hospital into academe appeared to provide an optimal solution. The fact was that many hospitals, freed of the necessity of expanding training for a wide array of AHP specialists and technicians, were agreeable to providing clinical work sites for the newly burgeoning college based programs.

Table 12.2, for 1975–76, shows the extent to which collegiate training of AHP had come to dominate both with respect to programs and graduates. Hospitals still continued to perform a training mission but in terms of graduates they accounted for only one out of every six.

Several additional facts: The 6,900 programs prepare students for 148 different occupations, mostly for entry-level assignments. The collegiate structure has 170,000 first-year places, for which they receive about 400,000 applications. Minorities account for about one in seven of the enrollees, most of whom (three out of four) are women.

The number of hospital programs with 35,000 graduates were heavily concentrated in clinical laboratory, radiologic technology, administration and planning, mental health, and dietetics.

The "Other nonmilitary" training institutions included in Table 12.2 refer primarily to vocational-technical schools, two-thirds public, one-third proprietary. The latter prepare students primarily for medical office assisting, dental assisting, nursing aid, dental laboratory, and medical laboratory, etc.

The military has long been a trainer of the personnel it needs to perform essential functions. But many who are trained to serve in military

Table 12.2   AHP-Training Structure

Setting	Institutions	Programs	Graduates
Collegiate, total	1,700	6,900	145,000
Noncollegiate, total	2,500	4,700	75,000
Hospitals	1,600	3,300	35,000
Other nonmilitary	900	1,300	20,000
Military	UNR	100	2,000
Total	4,200	11,600	220,000

Source: HEW Report III-2.

institutions leave after their initial tour of duty or after one or more reenlistments. Still relatively young, they need jobs after their return to civilian life. For those who were trained and employed in the military in health occupations who desire to find comparable jobs after discharge, the federal government has funded a series of "transition programs" to facilitate such conversion.

PROFESSIONALIZATION

Physicians learned a long time ago that they could advance their professional interests and at the same time help to advance their economic well-being through organizing themselves to exercise leadership over medical education, graduate training, hospital appointments, and to deal with other groups in society, governmental and nongovernmental. Small wonder, therefore, that AHP groups have sought to follow the same model by organizing themselves into associations, with an aim of exercising control via accreditation over the educational and training structures through which students must pass and of establishing systems for registration, certification, or, where indicated, licensing as a precondition for entrance into the field. However, the tight training structure of medical education with only about 126 schools in comparison to no fewer than 4,200 institutions involved in AHP training suggests that the medical pattern is not directly applicable.

Nonetheless, an older and better organized group such as the American Medical Technologists (AMT), established in 1939, is engaged in the following range of activities: registering medical laboratory personnel at three different levels—medical assistant, medical laboratory technician, medical technologist, for each of which the AMT has specified the required level of education and experience. Next, the AMT through an autonomous agency is involved in accreditation, which means that the agency assesses the quality of the preparatory programs and approved those that meet its standards. The AMT has, in addition to a national structure, a regional and state structure, which enables members to engage in educational, public information, representational, and similar activities. The AMT publishes a bimonthly journal that features primarily scientific articles of interest to the membership but that also devotes space to economic, political, and organizational developments. Since its organization forty-one years ago, AMT has certified over 30,000 individuals, but, as its president recently noted, there remain about "120,000 laboratory workers in the U.S. not certified by any agency."

A scanning of the *Health Careers Guidebook* (hereafter *Guidebook*),[2] calls attention to the multiple agencies that are involved in accreditation, examination, certification, and licensing. To stay with medical laboratory technicians and technologists: The AMA's Committee on Allied Health, Education, and Accreditation approves training programs. Upon graduation, however, the successful candidate can be certified by different organizations and in a minority of states, including Florida, Georgia, Pennsylvania, they must be licensed.

If one stands back from the pulling and hauling that goes on within the broad domain of AHP as to the goals of professionalization and the best ways of accomplishing training, certification, or licensing, one can identify the following underlying forces, several of which operate at cross purposes. As noted earlier, the functions to be performed by different groups of health workers from the physician to the assistant are subject to continuing change in response to the dynamism of medicine, the incentives for physicians to delegate routine responsibilities to others so as to free their time for more complex tasks, the differing patterns for organizing the performance of routine tasks within and outside of institutions depending on the volume of work and availability of trained personnel, the ambivalence of the AMA about professional goals for AHP, the realization on the part of the AMA leaders that they must not assume a dominating role, and the stake that many medical and surgical specialty groups have in structuring the conditions under which AHP assists them.

Although HEW has taken small steps now and again in the direction of setting national standards for educational institutions, competency examinations, and licensing regulations, the members of Congress, especially those from rural and low-income states, have seen to it that the status quo is altered, if at all, only at a rate at which institutions in their communities can accommodate. Nowhere is the gap between medical practitioners and AHP wider than in the arena of national standard setting.

JOBS AND CAREERS

In the *Guidebook* noted above, there are several pages of graphs which list a great many health occupations, indicating the years of education and training beyond high school graduation required for entrance into the field. Most assistants and many technicians, such as certified laboratory assistants and histological technicians, can qualify on the basis of one year's instruction. At the opposite extreme are specialist in blood bank technology, five years; medical social worker, six years; speech pathologist and audiologist, six years. In between, one finds physical therapist assistant, two years; dispensing optician, two years; radiation therapy technologist, two years; cytologist, three years; prosthetist, four years; orthotist, four years. Even if human capital theory cannot by itself account fully for differences in lifetime earnings, much of the variability in earnings among AHP workers that we will soon identify is linked to the time and expense that they have invested in their preparation.

The salary and career prospects of AHP are strongly affected by the following. The first is that the predominance of women in the field has a depressing influence on the salary structure. Discrimination against women in the labor market has been characteristic of our economy, and while recent legislation, administrative practices, and institutional arrangements have begun to shift in the direction of greater equity, women generally remain seriously disadvantaged with respect to salaries and promotional opportunities.

While there were a few years in the latter 1960s when many health care institutions found themselves shorthanded with respect to AHP, the responsiveness of the educational and training structures prevented significant long-term shortages from developing which in turn weakened the ability of AHP to bargain for substantial increases in salaries. A considerable number of AHP not employed in hospitals work for physicians in private practice. The physician is in a relatively strong bargaining position since he determines the qualifications of those whom he selects to assist him and the functions which he delegates, and his employees face difficulties in organizing to press their demands.

As noted earlier, one of the concomitants of the drive toward professionalization is the increasing control exercised by the more potent AHP organizations over their field, and the conditions of entrance and advancement. Each of the groups—assistants, technicians, technologists—seeks to build protective barriers, the consequence of which is to limit the occupational mobility open to members who are at a lower rung. While the American Medical Technologists have structured an occupational ladder that enables individuals at the bottom to advance through additional education, training, and experience, their approach is the exception. More often than not, both embryonic and established AHP professional associations place obstacles in the path of persons who seek to advance on the basis of experience by insisting that they scale specific educational hurdles which, for reasons of time and cost, many of the upwardly mobile are unable to accomplish.

While the acquisition of diplomas and degrees is definitely the preferred route to employment and advancement in some of the newer occupations, as well as in some of those that have been long established, opportunities exist for trading experience for education. To illustrate: biomedical equipment technician: "In some cases individuals with less than an associate degree may substitute experience for education requirements."[3]

POLICY CONSIDERATIONS

Before assessing the more important policy issues involving AHP currently on the nation's agenda or likely to be added in the near future, it may be useful to look back and sketch in broad outline what has been occurring on the policy front during the highly dynamic post-World War II era. Credit for coping goes first to the hospital sector, which early recognized that its only prospect for meeting its manpower requirements was through expanding its training activities.

The second principal contributor was state governments, which by the early 1960s were increasingly active in expanding their collegiate establishments, both at the junior and senior college level, which, sensitive to their students' vocational interests and goals, responded by instituting training opportunities for AHP occupations.

The federal government, at least in terms of its health manpower programming (HEW), was a latecomer. Its first modest appropriations date from 1966, and in the following thirteen years federal outlays for AHP totaled $276 million,[4] or slightly over $20 million a year for construction, training, special projects, and other designated objectives. The department's objectives were set out as follows:

- To assure an adequate supply
- To assure adequate quality
- To minimize costs of health services
- To increase opportunities for the disadvantaged
- To increase the effectiveness of education and training
- To optimize geographic and specialty distribution

In sketching the evolution of AHP one must also take note of the striking changes which occurred regarding the role of women in the labor force. Between 1950 and 1980 the proportion of women aged sixteen and over in paid employment increased from about one-third to over one-half. Women accounted for approximately three out of every five new job holders during these decades. The large inflow of women into the world of work during a period when the health care system was expanding rapidly was mutually supportive. Without the much enlarged supply of women workers, the health care industry could not have moved forward so rapidly. And the rapid expansion of health care created a large number of relatively attractive employment opportunities for many female job seekers.

The federal government, concerned over the significant shortage of physicians (estimated in the mid-1960s at 50,000) played a more active role in furthering the development of new training programs for physicians assistants (PAs) or physician extenders, the first effort having been initiated at Duke University in the mid-1960s. Federal officials saw in the physician assistant a rapid and cost-efficient way of responding to the physician shortage. It also early encouraged the specialty societies to experiment with using extenders and helped to finance programs for physicians assistants in pediatrics, urology, allergy, orthopedics, and surgery in addition to assisting the establishment and expansion of programs for physicians assistants in primary care. More recently it has centered its support on the latter making funds available for about forty such programs. Once the Washington officialdom decided (early 1970s) that the perennial physician shortage had been resolved, federal policy with respect to physicians assistants faced a dilemma. Why continue to train PAs in the face of a possible surplus of physicians?

It is difficult to see how the training of PAs can expand in the 1980s in the face of a substantially increased inflow of fully trained physicians. Some of the specialty societies, such as orthopedists, early concluded that the training of PAs was not desirable and terminated their programs. With the nurse leadership belatedly, but aggressively, pushing to expand the number of nurse practitioners the future role of the PAs becomes equivocal. Other issues that have never been adequately resolved affect the scope of practice of PAs when they are under the direct or indirect supervision of physicians and the reimbursement of their services under Medicare and Medicaid.

If one were forced to make a forecast of the future role of PAs it would be safer to assume that the training programs will shrink rather than expand and that among those currently employed as well as future graduates a significant minority will be lost through attrition. It is highly unlikely that PAs will have any significant effect on altering the pattern of delivering health care to the population as a whole.

This brief discussion of the future of PAs helps to point up a generic issue about the effective deployment of AHP. From the vantage of a health planner one can identify a great many settings where the substitution of less for more trained personnel under appropriate supervision would be cost reducing without loss of quality. But these opportunities do not turn into realities because of the self-interest of affected practitioners, systems of reimbursement, legal constraints on practice, consumer preferences, and the absence in many cases of organizational structures necessary to take advantage of such potential efficiencies and economies. To drive the last point home: Even in the federal establishment—the armed forces, the Veterans' Administration, the Public Health Service—there has been at best only modest progress in the effective utilization of AHP. There has been much talk about encouraging physicians to work with AHP as a "team," but the fact is that the organizational structures for the delivery of health care in the United States are basically antagonistic to the optimal utilization of AHP even under prepayment plans and more so under fee-for-service.

One must not jump to the conclusion, however, that in other countries where governments play a more active role in the health care system, one finds greater utilization of AHP. The study of Milton and Ruth Roemer (1978), provides interesting insights. The Roemers point out in their conclusions that, "In general . . . there are fewer categories and lesser relative numbers of their other allied health personnel in all the study countries than in the United States."[5]

Several AHP groups have sought in recent years to provide opportunities for individuals who have acquired additional knowledge and competence on the job and through training programs to demonstrate this through a written examination after which, if they are successful, they can move up the job and career ladder. But the development of good testing instruments is a difficult and expensive undertaking, and most AHP groups continue to place primary emphasis for certification and licensure on the completion of formal educational requirements.

The training of "narrow specialists" is dysfunctional for many smaller and even medium-sized hospitals where in the face of an explosion in technical procedures their need is for personnel trained to handle a variety of machines and competent to perform several technical procedures. Canada, according to the Roemers, is considering the training of such "critical care technologists" following upon its earlier combined training of laboratory and X-ray and physical and occupational therapists.[6]

The relationship between raising the requirements for credentialling and licensing and improvements in the quality of the service remains obscure. The presumption is deeply ingrained that better educated and trained persons perform better, make fewer mistakes, are alert to idiosyncratic results, know when they need to seek help. It is therefore discouraging to discover that the Center for Disease Control has found no improvement over a ten-year period in the quality of independent laboratories in bacteriology, parasitology, virology and only marginal improvements in other areas.[7]

The scale of future training efforts for AHP as well as for other health personnel should be subject to continuing scrutiny. The *Guidebook* takes a distinctly optimistic stance toward future openings in most AHP occupations. If the assumption of a marked slowdown in new fundings proves correct, it will be hard to justify its optimism about future manpower requirements.

A marked deceleration of new funds is likely to occur at the same time that the number of physicians per 100,000 is almost certain to increase by at least one-third (from 180 to 240) within a single decade. Physicians will be looking for ways to maintain their income in an environment in which dollars will be scarcer. It is likely that they will adopt a more restrictive stance toward others who see patients, especially PAs and nurse practitioners; they will seek to cut their overhead by reducing the number of helpers in their offices; and will return to doing work previously delegated to others.

To the extent that these forebodings are borne out, it is important for the states and the federal government to keep under close surveillance their appropriations for the training of AHP. There is no point in encouraging large numbers of young people to secure such training if the job market tightens appreciably. True, there will always be a reasonable number of replacement openings, and new breakthroughs in technology will create a demand for new specialists. But if containment rather than expansion in health care is the dominant theme, a cautionary training stance is indicated.

The last decade has seen gains in the education of AHP, especially through the establishment of schools of allied health personnel in large academic health science centers. Important innovations occurred involving new core curriculum, faculty improvement, broadened opportunities for clinical experience. The leadership of AHP emphasizes the need for continuing such efforts to strengthen the educational base.

The last important policy issue involves the changing relations of the federal government to the states, remembering that it is the states that have primary responsibility for the licensing of health personnel and for the regulation of health providers. Although the federal government made several feints in the 1970s toward setting national standards for the certification and/or licensing of selected groups of AHP, a critical review suggests that such intervention is premature. The several professional associations, working separately and cooperatively, should be encouraged to move in the direction of the national standard setting. To the extent that they are successful the next logical step is for the states to adjust their rules and regulations accordingly. If the efforts of nonprofit organizations and the states show reasonable progress there is no reason for the federal government to take the lead. If they fail there is little prospect of the federal government's succeeding.

The federal government has also made funding available in recent years to encourage professional associations to develop competency examinations so as to broaden the opportunity of those who have been trained mostly on the job. This is clearly a desirable approach if opportunities for improved mobility are not to be limited solely to individuals who have had access to educational programs.

A third sensible line of activity for the federal government is to continue, and possibly expand, the efforts which it helped to initiate to encourage a large group of AHP societies to work cooperatively toward improved examination and certification standards (National Commission for Health Certifying Agencies).

During the expansionary 1960s, not only in health but across the gamut of social policy, the dominant style in the United States was for professors, politicians, and public interest groups to identify unsolved problems and then to advocate new federal interventions aimed at removing the deficiencies that had been identified. One can, however, identify much that was not resolved, such as the optimal patterns of health manpower utilization, improved quality controls over the work performed by AHP, greater opportunities for occupational mobility for persons low on the totem pole, and reciprocity in licensing among the states.

These and other issues remain on the agenda. But if the recent past can provide guidance for the near future it should be that the accommodations between the supply and demand for AHP represent, unlike the case with physicians, a challenge to local institutions in which the principal actors have been and must continue to be individuals in search of jobs and careers; employers in search of workers; state governments involved in providing educational and vocational opportunities for the population; professional associations committed to improving the competence, status, and rewards of their members; and the federal government seeking to identify a limited number of frontiers where it can assume a leadership position. The future of AHP will depend more on the changes in structure of health care delivery than on the education and professionalization of the work force.

PART IV

Health Agenda

It has been made clear that our $400 billion health care system is flawed in many respects, and that the number of issues on the nation's health agenda exceed what any one analyst can hope to address. Several issues follow that address sequentially the role of research in medical progress, responses to disability and imminent death, and strategies for reform, introduced with some iconoclastic views in Chapter 13 and concluding with the "Coming Struggle for the Health Care Dollar" (Chapter 18).

Chapter 14 grew out of a request to me from the American Association of Medical Colleges (AAMC) that I determine how many dollars it would take to assure that American medicine remains in the forefront of modern therapeutics. My answer suggests that the sum is well within our reach.

Chapter 15 addresses an important subject that has received little attention: the potentials and limits of medical intervention once the physician broadens his focus from the reduction of disability to include estimates about the patient's future functionality.

Chapter 16 focuses on the care of dying and emphasizes that all that is subsumed under health care is not necessarily related to the control of disability and the improvement of functionality. Rather, a large proportion of all health care resources are directed to prolonging the life of the dying, a process which often inflicts pain and indignity on patients and their families rather than providing them with palliation and comfort.

Chapter 17 summarizes the advice I recently gave Congress with respect to the prospective deficit in the Medicare Trust Fund. The chapter makes a strong plea for a narrow search for more revenue rather than a comprehensive attack on the issue of containing health care costs. The country is not ready for the second issue, and in the interim the earlier gains that the elderly and the disabled have received from Medicare should be protected.

Chapter 18 advances the argument that in the years ahead there will be intensified struggles among physicians, between physicians and hospitals, between physicians and other health care providers for the increasingly constrained total dollars that will be available. The relatively sedate relations among the key parties that have prevailed over the past two generations are gone and are not likely to return.

13

Some Nonconventional Views

MORE PHYSICIANS DO NOT ASSURE GREATER ACCESS

Unlike most people in this country, I have never believed that we ever had a physician shortage. I wrote in the *New England Journal of Medicine* in 1960 that the question of the number of physicians and the question of access to the health care system were two different things, and we should not confuse them.[1] We did confuse them. We thought that if only we had more physicians, everybody would have access. I did not believe that then; I do not believe it now. So I have always been opposed to increasing the supply of physicians by Herculean efforts.

However, we are going to have a sudden big increase in the supply of physicians. It took us the last thirty years to move from 140 to 180 doctors per 100,000 population. We are now going to move from 180 to 240 in only ten years. This represents a 200 percent acceleration in the rate of increase. There is a figure that I helped to popularize: each new physician adds about $350,000 in costs per year to the system. Hence, more physicians mean higher costs. If we wanted to change this pattern, what steps could we take? A governmental plan could perhaps constrict the supply by subsidizing medical schools as they cut the size of their entering classes. But that will not happen for a long time.

THERE IS NO SIGNIFICANT MALDISTRIBUTION PROBLEM

I have never believed that we had a significant maldistribution problem, either by specialty or by geography. Dr. Linda Aiken and her colleagues have recently published the report of a Robert Wood Johnson Foundation

Originally published as "Some (Non-Conventional) Views on Health Care Reform," *Man and Medicine* **5**, 1980. Reprinted by permission.

study conducted with the University of Southern California.[2] They found
that of the 80 percent of the population that has a regular source of primary care 20 percent receives this care from a specialist. (This fact does
not appear to bother the authors—in my view correctly.) Primary care provided by specialists has to be included in estimates of primary care availability.

As far as geography goes, it stands to reason that, in an unequal society
with differentials in income, all resources will be differentially distributed—reflecting the fact that people and incomes are unevenly distributed. Therefore, there are many more physicians on Park Avenue than
in Harlem or Bedford-Stuyvesant. No one claims that this gives a satisfactory pattern of care, but the uneven distribution does not mean that
New York City has a geographic shortage of physicians.

THE "TEAM APPROACH" IS NO TEAM APPROACH

It is commonly held that what really makes for good medical care is the
"team approach." It is true that at the beginning of this century we had
one physician to two other members of the health team, and that now we
have something like one to fourteen. The real question about teamwork
in medicine is: Who has the power and who controls the process? I would
argue that the health team is not a team at all; it is a group of assistants,
largely dominated by the physician. The assistants are additive, not substi-
tutive. Even in a clinic like the Martin Luther King Clinic in the Bronx,
most of the paramedics are additive.[3] As long as there is money, it is easy
to add people to the team.

THE POOR ARE THE RECIPIENTS OF EXCESSIVE
MEDICAL INTERVENTION

The danger is not—as has been maintained—that the poor do not have
enough access to medical care. I submit that the opposite danger is the
real one; that is, since the advent of Medicare and Medicaid they have
had too much access and therefore have been subjected to too much medical intervention. Why are operation rates among the poor frequently
higher than among the non-poor? It is true that many of the poor may be
in need of surgery, but I believe that the number of operations has been
excessive. The presumption that encounters with the health care system
are necessarily good is, of course, one that is frequently counter to fact.

HEALTH CARE REFORM IS NOT AMONG
THE FIRST PRIORITIES OF THE POOR

Health care reform must be seen in relationship to other needed reforms.
I served as the long-term Chairman of the National Commission for

Employment Policy, and this gives me an informed perspective on the needs of the poor. The poor, when asked, do not put health care any- where near the top of their list of priorities. They want jobs, they want food, they want to get rid of the rats in their houses. They usually men- tion some fourteen priorities before they come to improved health care services. That does not mean that their health care is ideal, far from it.

NURSE PRACTITIONERS PROVIDE BETTER PRIMARY CARE TO THE POOR

When it comes to treating the poor, it makes eminently more sense to use the services of nurse practitioners than it does to try to force physicians to do what they have never done willingly anywhere in the world, including the Communist countries: to practice among the poor. I believe that phy- sicians and the poor do not, fundamentally, relate well. The poor do not like to ask physicians for favors; physicians do not like to treat the poor— unless, of course, they are suffering from an interesting disease in a teach- ing hospital. I think we can—and I so recommended to Alabama and other states—strengthen public nursing and nurse practitioners, so that with backup support from physicians and with transportation chits, we can provide good primary care to the poor. As a way to improve access to the system, this appears to me to be much the better approach.

PREVENTION IS NOT THE PANACEA IT IS CURRENTLY THOUGHT TO BE

It is often argued nowadays that we put too much money into therapeutic medicine and that we ought to put much more into prevention. I ask: What specific interventions are you talking about? All the prevention we know how to do is, basically, being done. (True, we do not get every last youngster at the right time for his immunizations.) Pap smears have prob- ably been effective in reducing deaths from cervical cancer. There is a role for prevention in averting the complications of hypertension. The National Institutes of Health are exploring ways of putting more effective hypertension control programs into place, and of finding and following the people who ought to be under treatment. But aside from these few interventions—early immunization, Pap smears, and hypertension con- trol—and aside from environmental protection, almost everything that has to do with prevention is embedded in personal behavior.

Personal behavior is a wholly different problem. We know we are not supposed to smoke, eat so much, be as inert as many of us are (though more and more of us are becoming involved in activities relating to keep- ing fit). In a democracy it is not easy to enforce behavior changes. In fact, in a free society, we may be obligated to permit some people to die early if they so prefer. It is not the government's job to tell them that they must prolong their lives by changing their behavior. Government could, however, do a better job at health education. About 85 percent of our young people stay in high school long enough to obtain a diploma; about one in four graduate from college. There is ample opportunity here to educate for health.

On the environmental front, there is great confusion between risks, real dangers, and aesthetics—and there is much that is simply aesthetic here. What we do not know about the real dangers is well worth knowing. We do know something about the risks. We will learn more in the years ahead as we struggle to make the environment substantially risk-free. In the absence of really effective ways of testing the thousands of new chemicals that come into use every year, we are only at the beginning in controlling the environment to any significant extent. It will be that way for a long time to come, and it will be a very rough game. I do not believe that it is realistic for us to expect that we can substantially reduce the health risks in the environment or make significant advances in preventive medicine in the near future. That does not mean that we do not have to work on these fronts; we do. But much of the "conventional wisdom" about the value of prevention is vastly exaggerated and does not hold up.

One must think broadly about the factors that influence health. In my opinion, the most significant contribution to the good health of the American people over the last ten years has been the Food Stamp Program. At the cost of a relatively few billions of dollars, we have largely eliminated malnutrition in this country.

OTHER NATIONS' HEALTH CARE SYSTEMS ARE NO BETTER THAN OURS

We are constantly reading about the wonderful health care systems that exist elsewhere in the world. As far as I know, none of them is any better than ours. Rudolf Meidner, the chief economist of the Swedish trade union movement told me, "For God's sake, if you come to Sweden, don't get sick on a weekend; and don't get sick in the months of June and July, because you'll never see a physician!"

Canada is at the moment the great model for health care delivery. But increasing numbers of Canadian physicians are leaving the national insurance plan and opting for private payment. And increasing numbers are coming south, almost one thousand last year. I have not yet heard of large numbers of physicians going north because it is such a wonderful system.

Cuba's health care system is also widely praised. But Cuba is not comparable to the United States; that small island has a wholly different economic and social structure. In Russia, the top bureaucracy has its own private physicians, private clinics, private hospitals. Outsiders cannot even get inside to look at them. One of the reasons that many Russian scientists want to emigrate to Israel or elsewhere is that they are deprived of access to this exclusive system, which is open only to the top bureaucracy. Everything is very special for the top people in Russia—everything from country estates to health care.

NATIONAL HEALTH INSURANCE, AS PROPOSED, IS AN EXPENSIVE FICTION

We have had national health insurance on our nation's agenda since 1912—one year after I was born. I have never believed that it was going to be passed. Something may be passed that will be called national health insurance, but I hope nobody will be fooled by the name. The Congressional Budget Office estimated several years ago that a comprehensive national health insurance plan would require, in terms of federal financing (not in terms of net total expenditures), something in the neighborhood of $100 billion dollars additional for the federal budget. What the net cost now would be, nobody knows.

Probably 15 percent of the population of this country is without any health insurance coverage, or with very inadequate coverage. But from the remaining 85 percent of the public, we do not hear very much by way of complaint. In a democracy in which the 85 percent outvotes the 15 percent, I see limited scope for helping the 15 percent not covered—if that means upsetting the entire system. All we can hope to do is to improve the extant system. And I think that we made, and will sometime in the future again make, modest efforts in that direction. Even conservatives in Congress have proposed bills aimed at providing protection against catastrophic illness and improving Medicaid coverage. But most of the poor and elderly will still have their infirmities and disabilities, even with a little better access to care.

COST CONTAINMENT IS NOT IMPOSSIBLE

Cost containment is a difficult issue. Most people who write about it contend that because the health industry does not follow a competitive model, health costs cannot be controlled; the consumer does not have any power of deterrence and therefore the system spends too much money. There is a modicum of truth to this, but only a modicum. I can guarantee that we will not have a perpetual increase in health costs at 50 percent above the Consumer Price Index. This may happen for a few more years, but it will not happen indefinitely. The American public has no intention of investing more and more of its disposable income in medical care. People want to travel, to eat out more often, to provide their offspring with a good education. Medical care is not the beginning and end of everything. We may go from 10 to 12 percent, maybe even to 15 percent, of the gross national product—but that is all.

It will take a while to bring a large and amorphous sector such as the health care system under control, but we are slowly putting the brakes on. State rate-setting commissions, Blue Cross, industry, and the trade unions are beginning to move. Hospital days of care in New York City hospitals are now below 500 per 1,000 a year. That is the rate that obtains in a reasonably efficient health maintenance organization.

Until recently, industry and labor, the two major purchasers of insurance, played no active role. They are now becoming interested, and for a simple reason: the annual health insurance cost for a worker at General Motors (just under $3,000 a year) is more than the cost of the steel that goes into a Chevrolet. At this scale, neither the employer nor the union can remain indifferent. One must, however, be aware that there is a danger in the new interest of business and labor in cost containment. The two may well collaborate in writing contracts at the lowest cost (based on experience rating), leaving the community vulnerable. We have seen what happens when Medicare and Medicaid cut corners on reimbursement: hospitals must find other ways to cover their costs.

Health care today is a very big industry—$360 billion and over 7 million jobs. Much of what transpires has more to do with employment and income than with health. Real economies are made, not by closing excess surgical and medical beds, but only by closing entire hospitals. If one closes a hospital, one takes admitting privileges away from physicians and jobs away from workers. This is not easy, as we found out in the recent closure program in New York City. Neither the British nor the Russians, both of whom operate a national health system, find closing hospitals easy either. The process could be eased. Preferential hiring would have to be provided for all discharged workers; alternative staff assignments for physicians would have to be arranged. Complicated, yes, but not impossible.

The question of what one gets by spending more on medical care is an interesting one. I have argued in the past that if one is born healthy, has good genes, receives one's innoculations as scheduled, and does not have the bad luck to be hit by a truck, one has little need for medical care until one begins to disintegrate, at which point the system is not able to help very much. The system cannot provide good genes or good luck. What it can provide is some kind of relief from pain, occasionally a life-saving intervention, and mostly reassurance. Half of all ambulatory care visits end more or less as follows: "Go home and take an aspirin." If we ever learn how to use the telephone intelligently, we could save a great many visits.

PREPAID MEDICAL PLANS ARE NO SOLUTION

I am not a believer in the significance of medical cooperatives or prepaid plans—HMOs, IPAs, or any other such set of initials. They promise little change in the health care delivery system. In New York City, we have one of the oldest prepaid plans: HIP. It has stagnated. And Group Health in Washington, which is an old cooperative, suffered a physicians' strike in 1978 because the specialists were dissatisfied with an annual salary of over $80,000. They wanted the right to engage in private practice in addition. While I expect that HMOs will grow, I expect them to grow slowly, because I do not think that they are the answer, either from the point of view of most consumers or from that of many providers. Many physicians find it difficult to work in that kind of structure; most consumers do not want to have their choices restricted. The whole trend in consumer behavior goes the other way—to more, not fewer, choices.

HEALTH CARE CANNOT BE BASED ON
A COMPETITIVE MODEL

The Federal Trade Commission is seeking to establish competition as the guiding principal in the health care system. If there is anything that by definition is a quasi monopoly, it is a hospital. If there is any validity to the concept of a professional, then a physician by virtue of his specialized training is capable of making judgments about health care that other people cannot. How does one, in the face of these elementals, turn health care into a competitive model? I appreciate that the FTC is trying to eliminate the most exploitative practices of various physicians' groups that have sought to protect themselves from all outsiders. I have no objection to such action. But many with new religion in Washington do not really know how the health field functions.

What observations underlie these non-conventional views on health care reform? The first is that services generally, both in the private market, and, particularly, in the governmental market, are very hard to deliver effectively. If they have to be delivered to the mass of the population, it is an even more complex task. We have been supporting public education in the North in this country for close to two hundred years—and still at least 20 percent of all youths and 40 percent of youths in the ghettos leave school functionally illiterate. After two hundred years of experience, we do not know how to assure that everyone learns to read and write. In comparison to two other major public services—education and criminal justice—the health sector looks pretty good. It is not in fact very good; all government services are hard to deliver, as are many services in the market; witness the long lines of people in banks waiting at the teller's window, and the number of billing errors made by department stores.

Second, the federal government has no useful experience in the direct delivery of services to the public. One—the postal service—government did so badly that the task was shifted to a special non-Cabinet organization. The only other service that the federal government shares with the states is the Job Service. The Job Service succeeds in placing only about 20 percent of all people who obtain jobs in the course of a year, and these mostly into low-paying, short-term employment. Anybody who thinks that the health care system can be modified by a wave of the congressional hand, and that delivery of good services can thus be assured to 235 million people throughout the United States, is not being realistic. Health care delivery demands local resources, local institutions, local practitioners, and an effective relationship between providers and the people who want and need the services.

It must always be remembered that the delivery of any service, especially a complicated service, involves a reciprocal relationship between the provider and the consumer. Health care cannot be improved without the active participation of the consumer. It is like education: you cannot educate someone unless he participates. If a physician prescribes for a patient, and the patient does not follow instructions, the system breaks down, no matter how competent the physician. We know that the slippage between the physician giving orders and the patient following those orders is substantial. The reciprocal relationship of patient and physician is critically important and must be kept in view in all discussions about reforming the health care system.

I will conclude by noting that most of the conventional ideas about the reform of the health care system are, in my opinion, unrealistic. The people who advance them are generally naive about how the system really operates. They have little understanding of who holds the power and less understanding of what the consumer will settle for. I believe that we should try to identify the gravest defects in the extant system and seek incremental improvements. A total overhaul is neither indicated nor feasible.

How good—or how bad—is our health care system? The answer must be given in terms of other service systems. On that basis, not too bad, but it could be better.

14

Medical Progress: The Dollar Cost

The Stanford health economist Victor Fuchs noted some years ago that physicians usually hold their meetings without the help of an economist. However, when medicine faces difficult social or economic problems, an economist is included in the roster of speakers. What can we conclude, then, when the Association of American Medical Colleges (AAMC) presents two economists in two days at its plenary sessions other than that those who have arranged the program believe that American medicine is entering upon perilous times?

There is, of course, an alternative interpretation. If two economists are invited and they do not agree, then physicians can reach the not unreasonable conclusion that while they may be uncertain about where the system is heading, economists are equally unsure about what lies ahead. I have high regard for Professor Uwe Reinhardt of Princeton University, who addressed the preceding plenary session, but it is necessary that I clarify the differences between us on three major counts.

First, Professor Reinhardt believes that the substantial federal budgetary deficits, which will amount to almost $200 billion annually for the next several years, will not derail the current economic recovery. Next he estimates that the U.S. economy will continue to grow until the end of the century at a rate that will enable the health care system to utilize, absolutely and relatively, a higher proportion of the nation's annual output and still leave the consumer with more disposable income for nonmedical consumption. Third, he believes that whether or not more funds are funneled into medical research and development is a matter of "taste." The American public, he says, will have the option of continuing to subsidize

Originally published as "Medical Progress: How Much Money Will It Take?" *Journal of Medical Education* 59 (367–72), May 1984. Reprinted by permission.

farmers at the current $20 billion per annum and/or invest more in medical research and development programs.

It may be a matter of generational differences, but a $200 billion annual deficit seems more of a threat to me than to Professor Reinhardt. Moreover, while he may be right in anticipating a sustained period of U.S. economic growth with substantial increases in total real output, the alternative prospect of major disruption of the international financial and trade systems cannot be dismissed out of hand. Finally, resort to the concept of taste as a determinant of how many dollars will flow into medical research and development is equivocal. It was President Reagan's taste to authorize the National Institutes of Health (NIH) budget for 1984 at a level of $400 billion below the figure that suited the taste of the Congress and the medical leadership, and the latter won.

We two economists share many values and preconceptions, but our appraisals of the present and forecasts of the future differ. Thus, what follows is my interpretation of the dollar dimension of medical progress, the role of nonmonetary factors in the equation, and a few suggestions for public policy which flow from the analysis.

PROPER CONTEXT

The following few figures will help to put the question of money in its proper context. In 1950 the total research and development budget of the United States amounted to 1 percent of the annual output of goods and services; that is, the nation was investing very little in research and development.[1] The medical research budget was 1/20th of this 1 percent. Thus, the medical research budget amounted to 1/20th of 1 percent of the gross national product (GNP) in 1950.

Dr. Julius Krevans spoke of the great explosion in biomedical knowledge that erupted in the post-World War II era.[2] But since significant gains in medical therapeutics had been made in the late 1940s and early 1950s, researchers were using a knowledge base that had been supported by less than 1/20th of 1 percent.

Dr. Robert Petersdorf's reference to the role of Alan Gregg in leveraging changes in medical education and research with relatively few Rockefeller Foundation dollars should be a further reminder that the relationship between dollars and medical progress is not as simple and direct as some people believe.[3]

Against this background of earlier modest investments in medical research and development, both absolutely and relatively, let us consider the range of outlays in the succeeding decades. Throughout the 1960s, we spent not 1 percent but roughly 3 percent of the GNP (in constant dollars) for research and development. And although there was a significant decline in the mid-1970s, investment in research and development at present still preempts about 2.4 percent of a much larger GNP, two and one-half times its postwar base.[4] Medical research and development is up from 1/20 to 3/10 of 1 percent, which represents a sixfold increase in three decades.

So far, we have considered only percentage changes on a rapidly expanding base, and these are difficult comparisons to grasp. Let us now shift focus to what happened in terms of dollar outlays.

In 1950 we spent on medical research and development about $160 million from all sources—government, private, and philanthropy. This year the total is in the neighborhood of $9.5 billion. When inflation is taken into account, the increase is reduced from about sixtyfold to fifteenfold— still quite an impressive gain.

Of particular interest to the AAMC is the proportion of medical research and development outlays that have gone to higher education—to the universities, colleges, and medical schools. Of the $160 million total in 1950, somewhat less than one-third, circa $50 million, went to academic health centers and universities. Today, the total is in the neighborhood of $3.5 billion.

There is no simple and sensible way to answer the question of how much money it will take to assure a continuing rapid rate of medical progress. But the foregoing figures should make one point clear. The American public, through Congress and industry, has not been niggardly in investing in medical research. Some might counter that medical research could have made use of still more money. Yes and no. The key question is: Would funneling more money into health research have been sound policy?

DECLINE OF MEDICAL RESEARCH

A recent publication of the AAMC[5] sets forth the following arguments, among others, to conclude that in the past decade or so there has been an underfunding of medical research.

1. In real dollar terms, the appropriations for the National Institutes of Health have been stable since the early 1970s. This means that there have been no funds available for growth despite the fact that the number of medical school graduates has been increasing.

2. The juxtaposition of stable dollars and an expanding supply of potential researchers points to the underutilization of the available capacity.

3. The number of new and competitive projects recommended to the NIH for funding and the declining proportions that have been funded are prima facie evidence that medical research is being underfunded.

4. Over the last decade or so, there has been a reversal in the proportions of post-doctoral researchers supported by the NIH who have an
M.D. degree and those with Ph.D.s. In the late 1960s, M.D.s exceeded
Ph.D.s by a wide margin; currently, Ph.D.s outnumber M.D.s by a ratio
of 2 to 1.

There is no need to counter these arguments by stipulating that a problem may not exist in recent trends in funding, but the following elements
must be weighed before the pessimistic conclusion of a decline in American medical research is accepted. Let us consider in turn each of the pro-
positions cited above.

1. Between 1950 and 1963, which was the heyday of federal expenditures for medical research, appropriations for the NIH increased at the
rate of almost 25 percent per annum, compounded. The theory of com-
pound interest should have served as a reminder that this trend could not
continue. Since 1963 the increase in real dollars has averaged around 3 to
4 percent with most of the gains predating 1973. The difference between a
3 to 4 percent rate of increase over a twenty-year period and a 25 percent
annual rate is about sevenfold; this means that had the NIH appropriations not been severely moderated, federal appropriations in 1983 would
have been of the order of $28 billion, not $4 billion. It is possible that the
latter figure is not optimal. But nobody will contend that the higher figure
or any approximation of it would be appropriate.

2. I was a young Ph.D. entering academic life in the mid-1930s, and I
can state that it was not assumed in those times that society would provide funding for every young person who had the ability and desire to
pursue research. And there was surely no obligation for our society to
assure such persons a stable and secure career.

3. On the basis of personal experience as a member of two advisory
councils of the NIH, I can state that whether it is necessary, or even desirable, to fund half of the approved projects is debatable. In some research
areas such a criterion may be sensible but not necessary in all.

4. There are surely different ways to interpret the declining ratio of
M.D.s to Ph.D.s among the new researchers. One approach is to place the
blame on an insufficiency of dollars flowing into medical research. But
there are other, more apposite explanations. These would include the
aging of the faculties of medical schools, which precludes the achievement
of tenure by many of the young researchers. In 1968 only one in five
faculty members was above 48 years of age; the estimate for 1990 is one
in two. Under these unfavorable conditions, it is not surprising that many
talented young physicians are thinking twice about opting for an
academic career. An economist would also point out that the differentials
in pay and perquisites might be assessed differently by physicians and

Ph.D.s. And a skeptic might question whether a clinical researcher without a doctorate in one of the core disciplines is adequately prepared for a research career in the decades ahead.

These formulations by themselves do not refute the claim that medical research in America is in decline, but they go a long way toward suggesting that the supporting arguments are not definitive.

SOME NONMONETARY CONSIDERATIONS

The questions should be raised, even though the answer will not be readily forthcoming, whether and to what extent medicine can move ahead without reference to the rate of progress in the core disciplines. Abraham Pais' marvelous biography of Albert Einstein, which centers around the origins of his ideas as well as their impact, demonstrates unequivocally what we know but tend to forget, namely the interdependency among the sciences. The equivocal results of targeted research is a further reminder of this basic truth when the problem is new understanding and not the application of existing knowledge.

In the late 1950s, in testimony before the Joint Atomic Energy Committee of the Congress, I stated that there were dangers in having too much money chasing too few talented researchers. The excessive funding at that time merely encouraged the proliferation of enterpreneurial professors who enhanced their ties to their peers but who had little identification with their schools. The lack of cooperation among medical school faculty members in confronting the wide range of issues which they must address, from revising the undergraduate curriculum to determining the size of residency programs, can be traced in large measure to the dysfunctional consequences of long-term liberal research funding.

My associate, George Vojta, executive vice president of Bankers Trust, and I are just completing a book, titled *Beyond Human Scale: The Large Corporation at Risk*, which contains a chapter on The Golden Age of the U.S. Corporation. We point out that it was a gross misunderstanding to assume, as many did in the 1950s and 1960s, at home and abroad, that the U.S. corporation had found the key through management sophistication to perpetual growth and profitability. A large part of its success resulted from the fact that it had the field for itself until Germany and Japan reentered the market.

The leaders of American medicine may have fallen into a similar trap. They have come to believe—and their colleagues abroad have reinforced their judgment—that it was the liberal financing of biomedical research that catapulted U.S. medicine into the lead. Without denying that such financing helped to speed the advance of U.S. medicine, we must admit that we looked better than we really were because all of the major competitors had been knocked out of the ring as a result of Hitler and the devastation of World War II.

On a related point of perspective, I have never accepted the views of Illich, LaLonde, and other critics of therapeutic medicine who claim that since mortality rates have declined only modestly, most of the expenditures for research and therapeutics result in little other than medical empires and an affluent profession. The late Walsh McDermott made more sense when he argued that the touchstone of medical progress is found not only in the decline of mortality rates but also in improvements in the quality of life which result from hip replacements, the removal of cataracts, the control of hypertension, and much more.

If McDermott's criteria are accepted, the hubris of the medical profession should be moderated by the realization that in the three decades following 1940 the expected years of life for an American man aged 65 or older were extended from 12 to 14 and for a woman of the same age from 13.5 to 18 years. A successful research attack on cardiovascular-renal diseases would add 11.5 years of life at age 65.[6]

CONCLUDING OBSERVATIONS

I first want to compliment the AAMC for performing its job so well. As an economist who is acquainted with the budgetary process in Washington, I find it impressive that Congress raised the President's budget for medical research by $400 million. This is no small accomplishment in a year when the Congress is on a tight leash.

In a recent article, Dr. Petersdorf presented the multiple reasons why he considers the academic health centers to be at serious risk and the urgent and large scale repairs that are required to assure their survival and productivity.[7] To understand the magnitude of the trouble they face, we need only call attention to the fact that at present a high proportion—about one-third—of the income of all major teaching hospitals comes from Medicare and Medicaid, and unless action is taken, the Medicare Trust Fund will be out of money by the end of the decade and will incur a deficit of $300 billion by 1995.[8]

To add to these ominous signs, graduate medical education is financed almost exclusively by reimbursements for patient care; the Advisory Committee for Social Security has recommended that all alternative sources of funding be explored so that this burden may be removed from the backs of patients.

It is no longer adequate to pose the question of whether the American people want good medical care. Of course they do. In fact, they want more, not less. The country continues to have a love affair with medicine, but it would like to cut out the roses and the expensive dinners while it continues to enjoy the pleasures that come with the relationship. In fact, the opinion survey reports disclose that the only group that the American public continues to hold in high esteem is physicians.

This respect and admiration, garnered over decades and generations, is to be cherished and protected, not squandered. The medical profession cannot maintain this unique and valuable relationship with the public by insisting that it is the sole guardian of the medical commons.

Ours is a democracy, and in a democracy the voters are interested not only in the quality of the health care delivery system but also in its efficiency and equity. If the medical profession continues to ignore questions of efficiency and equity, it stands to lose its credibility in the years to come when the dollar squeeze will most probably worsen. Unless the profession indicates that it is concerned about these values and is willing to make adjustments in its own behavior, it will risk the loss of its special relationship with the American people.

Congress is getting increasingly restive about what many of its members believe to be the excessive incomes of physicians. It is possible that an early piece of legislation aimed at the financial reform of Medicare will include a provision that physicians who treat Medicare patients will have to accept assignments or have their fees frozen. It is not too early for the AAMC to decide whether it will fight or acquiesce to such a congressional initiative.

In reaching a position on this and related issues, the AAMC might want to review with care the article by Roe on the usual, customary, and reasonable (UCR) system of paying physicians.[9] The argument and the conclusions cannot be dismissed as the work of an ill-informed economist.

A profession that commands the loyalty and respect of the public at large has a responsibility to help educate that public about the potential and limitations of modern medicine. Americans have never found it easy to accept death as an ineluctable fact of the human condition. Hence, they look to physicians to prolong their lives, even when the prospects of success are minimal. Physicians may need help from the clergy and the judiciary, as well as from the political leadership, in helping the public think and act more realistically about the terminal months and years of life. But unless physicians play a leading role, the public will continue to spend huge sums, suffer excessive pain, and face continuing disappointment.

There is one more task which, if skillfully pursued and carried out, could help the medical research community to solve its problem of inadequate funding. Dr. James Shannon noted in 1970 that, with Medicare and Medicaid on the books, liberal congressional funding for the cutting edge of medicine, education, and research was in jeopardy. Politicians always favor current services to the electorate over expenditures for new knowledge that may yield benefits in the future.

But there is a way to turn Shannon's pessimistic observation around. Currently, the national medical research budget is slightly below $10 billion out of a GNP of $3.5 trillion, of 3/10 of 1 percent. Surely, Congress would be willing to increase this small percentage if the medical leadership would offer to help constrain the total outlay for health care services, which totalled about $360 billion, or roughly 10.5 percent of the GNP, in 1983. The medical leadership can do this by playing a leading role in formulating recommendations aimed at reductions in medical school enrollments, in altering fee schedules for physicians, in slowing the rate of new costly half-way technology, and in helping to shift the delivery of health care from acute hospitals to ambulatory settings and home care.

If the leadership of academic medicine helps the Congress and the public to restrain the costs of the total health care delivery system, it could expect that its requests for additional funds for research would be met, even exceeded.

15

Disability and Functionality

This analysis addresses three interrelated themes. The first is the concept of disability and we will seek to clear up some of the conceptual fuzziness that attaches to it; the second identifies a limited number of issues that call for early assessment and action; the third points directions for improved public policies.

Several paradoxes overhang the subject of disability. The epidemiologists have emphasized that millions of Americans suffer from disabilities and chronic diseases which restrict partially or totally the lives of the afflicted. At the time when therapeutic medicine has been marching from one victory to the next, relatively little attention has been paid to disabled and chronically ill persons. Another paradox is suggested by the widespread belief that the increasing number of sick and disabled elderly will soon be flooding the nation's hospitals while the spokesmen for the elderly have been arguing that Medicare must be revised in favor of providing more ambulatory services.

Another paradox is imbedded in the attitudes and behavior of many physicians who believe that their task of diagnosing correctly and treating effectively the physical ailments of the patients who present themselves is difficult enough. Others believe that they must consider the total circumstances of the patient before deciding on a plan for therapy.

Another is grounded in the role of some sophisticated patients who recognize that some risk always attaches to medical treatment and who believe that they should include this factor in deciding whether and what type of therapy they are willing to undergo.

Originally published as "Disability and Functionality," The First Spaulding Memorial Lecture, Spaulding Rehabilitation Hospital, Massachusetts General Hospital, 1984. Reprinted by permission.

A striking recognition of this last consideration was recently provided in some remarks of the Administrator of the Health Care Financing Administration, Carolyne Davis, who explained that patients would be major beneficiaries of the new DRG system. Shorter stays in the hospital would reduce the risk of infection, would make them less likely subjects for unnecessary surgery, and they would have a better chance of avoiding an iatrogenic drug reaction.

In the face of these uncertainties, disagreements, and paradoxes, efforts at concept clarification hold promise of shaping understanding of the relationship of disability to functionality within the context of medical practice, today and tomorrow.

A good place to begin is to emphasize that many of life's most serious disabilities are not grounded in illness or injury but stem from societal or personal factors such as inadequate education, unemployment, low earnings, discrimination, and victimization. The medicalization of all ills is a disservice to both the individual under stress and to the society which seeks to assist him. Although people under stress often develop somatic complaints which require attention, it is unlikely that medical treatment alone will restore them to a satisfactory level of functioning.

A tendency to excessive medicalization can result in faulty policies with ominous consequences as was demonstrated by our experience in World War II. The military mistakenly relied on psychiatrists (often trained in ninety days!) to judge the suitability of selectees for service and also to judge whether servicemen who collapsed under stress should be retained or discharged. About 2.5 million young men out of a pool of about 16 million—1 in 6—were adjudged to be "ineffective" and were either rejected for or prematurely discharged from military service.

While most servicemen who were separated prematurely because of "psychoneuroses" or some similar diagnosis left with honorable discharges and often with small pensions, Private Slovak in administrative, not medical, channels ended up before a firing squad because he had insisted that the Army could not *force* him to fight.

A reaction to "overmedicalization" set in about fifteen years ago with the nihilistic attacks on modern therapeutics from Ivan Illich and the critical murmurs of some epidemiologists who believed that the elaborate structure of modern medicine was contributing little to the increasing longevity which they considered the best measure of effectiveness. And Marc LaLonde, the Canadian Minister of Health in the early 1970s, recommended that public expenditures be redirected from therapeutics to prevention of illness. If illness and injury were prevented there would clearly be little need for an ever more elaborate system of therapeutics. Unfortunately, LaLonde failed to specify just what a society could do to reduce disabilities so that the acute medical care system could be radically shrunk.

And the epidemiologists who looked to increases in longevity as the touchstone of the success of modern medicine ignored the equally important issue of the quality of life to which modern medical advances had contributed so much, from the prevention of blindness through cataract and other ophthalmic surgery to renewed mobility for persons who had fractured hips, to radiologic and chemotherapeutic control of selected cancers.

The elderly have been the main but not the only beneficiaries of the advances of modern medicine. The substantial increases in the number of older persons, particularly those over 80 and even 85, have raised questions about how our society will be able to cope with even larger numbers of disabled and infirm elderly. Some observers believe that our acute hospitals will soon be clogged with older patients and that we will have to double the capacity of our nursing homes.

The elderly certainly suffer from more chronic illnesses and as they age they become more frail. But to believe that most elderly are disabled, unable to live independently, and need large amounts of medical care is wrong. Many of the problems of the elderly reflect personal, not health problems: loss of job, loss of income, loss of spouse, loss of friends, loss of status. Although an increasing number need to be institutionalized usually because of a combination of senility, incontinence, and the absence of family supports, the vast majority of the older elderly, those over 85, live normal if restricted lives in their own communities and die while they are living in their own homes.

One more aspect of disability warrants clarification. In Western societies, illness and disability offer the individual a legitimate excuse for not working and supporting himself. Consequently, the ways in which a society deals with disability often contributes to its prevalence. Many sick or disabled persons learn to "exploit" their condition. In my student days at Heidelberg it was said that many senior professors had developed or held onto minor illnesses in order to achieve better control of their lives and provided excuses for avoiding the many demands on their time and energy. Many of these "disabled" persons lived into their eighties and a few into their nineties!

The complexity of the relationship between disability and functionality is best illustrated by reference to Franklin Delano Roosevelt. Stricken with polio in the prime of his life and never again able to stand unassisted, FDR functioned as Governor and as four-term president during two of the country's major crises—the Great Depression and its aftermath and World War II. Family, wealth, emotional support from his wife and his mother, and a strong personal drive for a leadership role enabled FDR to surmount a condition that would have justified his withdrawal from all forms of active participation. His life should remind us that the consequences stemming from even severe disability often depend on both

the emotional resilience of the individual and on his economic circumstances.

Three conclusions emerge from the foregoing effort at concept
clarification. The first is a reminder that the treatment of disability should
seldom be seen as exclusively "medical." Personal and societal considerations are always present and frequently dominate. Second, while sophisticated medicine can contribute substantially to the reduction and even
elimination of severe disabilities, its scope is narrowed as the patient
approaches the end of his life. Finally, we must be more discriminating in
our assessment of the amount and severity of disability and chronic illness
among the elderly. Most of the elderly, even the older elderly, do not
suffer from major disabilities that prevent their being able to live independent lives.

Our second task is to identify a number of issues about disability and
functionality that warrant early assessment and action. The first can be
designated as the "demographic" issue. The numbers of the elderly are
increasing both absolutely and relatively and this trend is particularly pronounced among the older elderly, that is, persons over 85. At the same
time it should be noted that the major demographic change will not occur
until around 2010 when the post-World War II baby-boom population
reaches retirement age. The larger number of the elderly, including a
larger number of frail elderly women living alone, precipitates the issue of
developing alternatives to institutionalization since most elderly would
prefer to continue living in the community and the costs of expanding
nursing homes are high.

A second issue involves a reconsideration of the use of the full
armamentarium of therapeutic medicine for patients who at birth, in their
middle years, and near the end of their lives have little promise of obtaining or regaining functionality for independent living or for meaningful
participation. From Baby Doe to the brain-damaged accident victim, to
the elderly person suffering from incurable cancer, several questions command attention: the right of the individual (or his surrogate) to choose an
earlier over a delayed death; the physical and emotional costs to patient
and family of decisions that form one or the other outcome; the challenge
of society's investing more and more of its resources in the moribund.

A third issue involves the criteria for judging societal investments aimed
at reducing disability and improving functionality. Consider the following
three cases. Years ago the vocational rehabilitation system in the State of
California provided a private tutor from first grade through college for
each blind student at an estimated cost in current dollars of close to
$400,000. The question is not whether such students could profit from this
opportunity but whether taxpayers should be required to underwrite such
an expensive program.

.Or consider the recent harsh words traded by the Mayor of New York City and the Governor about the remodeling of subway kiosks to provide access for the handicapped. Mayor Koch insisted that even after the remodeling the handicapped would still be unable to use underground transit and the odds are that he is right to call the plan a sentimental waste of funds.

There is considerable support, especially among spokesmen for the elderly, for the expansion of Medicare to provide a full panoply of home and community health, financial, and social work services. But most advocates ignore the fact that the individual and his or her family are now covering about 70 percent of these costs and if government were to assume them, it would result in a major tax on younger persons.

With a prospective deficit of $300 billion in its trust fund, the Medicare program must be revised by cutting entitlements, raising additional revenues, or both. The administration wants to have the beneficiaries enlarge substantially their copayments when they are hospitalized. Many Democrats prefer to have a surcharge placed on the income-tax paying elderly who enroll in Supplementary Medical Insurance. Others (Kennedy-Gephardt) are in favor of a major overhaul which would place a ceiling on all federal outlays for health care. The only certainty is that one or more of the foregoing actions, and probably still others, cannot be delayed.

The fifth issue relates to the alternative employment and income transfer policies which can have powerful impacts on the disabled and the elderly. Spurred by their Calvinist tradition, the Dutch have established workshops for their disabled in the belief that every person must be afforded the opportunity to engage in useful work. On the other hand, the Dutch and most other West Europeans have been encouraging retirement at age 60 and in special situations even earlier. In the United States, we have moved in the opposite direction to raise the retirement age or to remove age as a factor in employment. The welfare and well-being of the disabled and the elderly will be clearly affected by the decisions which our society reaches with respect to these social policies. The linkages may not always be evident but they exist.

Since disability is an important arena for health and social policy the preceding discussion of the five issues selected for brief inspection make or reinforce one critical point: we need more understanding of the complex nature and ramifications of disability and more assessments and explorations of how best to respond to it. As some contribution to this we now present some possible directions for public policy.

In tackling the problem of the Medicare Trust Fund deficit, Congress has a choice between "patching things up" or undertaking a major overhaul of Medicare and also of the entire American health care system by seeking to cap total outlays. My view is that the many gains provided by Medicare for the elderly and the disabled should be preserved, both the range of entitlements and the present levels of copayments, except for the affluent elderly who should be required to pay more. I have urged the Congress to find new tax revenues to reestablish the solvency of the Trust Fund and to avoid undertaking an overhaul of the entire U.S. health care system since the public and the providers are not ready for it.

The one arena where fundamental change is urgently required relates to "dying care." The reason that the elderly who comprise about 11 percent of the population use 30 percent of health care services is that most persons who die are elderly and as individuals approach death they make use of a great amount of care, particularly in the last sixty days of life. Physicians, politicians, and the public must engage in a broad dialogue about appropriate policies of care during the "last days of life." The opinion survey results indicate that the time is ripe for more discussion and early action.

Most informed persons advocate a vast expansion of community and home health care to reduce the flow of the increasing numbers of elderly into nursing homes. We must remember our lack of success with deinstitutionalizing the mentally ill as well as the substantial costs of caring for the bedridden in the absence of adequate family support. New York City spends close to half a billion dollars a year on home health care to enable 30,000 poor persons to avoid institutionalization. I am reasonably certain that we need to expand home care and community support services but we probably cannot avoid building additional nursing home capacity in any case.

One recent notable development has been the growth of self-help groups which now number over 5 million members, overwhelmingly persons suffering from disabilities and chronic illness. These people can learn a lot from each other in their search for mutual support. DeWitt Stetten, Jr.'s article in the *New England Journal of Medicine* some years ago was a powerful indictment of the gap between the advice and help that the disabled require and the knowledge and assistance that physicians provide.

Congress has been concerned periodically with the problem of "orphan drugs," those drugs which are vitally needed by only a few patients. How can it encourage the pharmaceutical industry to undertake the R&D to find new drugs for conditions that afflict only small numbers of patients? I suspect that the disability arena presents an "orphan technology" challenge. How can we stimulate the medical supply and appliance industry to shift some of its focus from in-hospital to out-of-hospital needs of the disabled? We must do more to add to the functionality of the non-institutionalized disabled.

The segmentation of the health care system has made it difficult and often impossible for physicians, particularly surgeons, to follow up on their interventions and to learn of their effectiveness in altering both the length and quality of their patients' lives. Many acute hospitals are currently looking to vertical integration as a preferred way to assure their economic future. I question how much money they will make from running nursing homes, home care programs, hospices. But I suspect that if their staffs have the opportunity to observe and treat their discharged patients over months and years, we will make significant gains in treating patients with chronic illness.

We need to focus more on enlarging the scope of public intervention through the use of police power to reduce many of the causes of disability from mandating seatbelts to tightening controls over drunken driving. Again, in a period of severe federal deficits it is hard to understand the logic—not the politics—of Congress' having agreed to cut back the tax on cigarettes from 16¢ to 8¢ a pack.

Even more difficult to institute are actions directed to more effective social interventions to reduce discrimination, poverty, child abuse, access to drugs which take a large toll in morbidity and preventable deaths. The homicide rate for young black males in New York City stands at 70 per 100,000, forty and fifty times the rate for West European countries.

Finally if I had to put forward a single societal intervention that holds the greatest promise of the enhancement of the functionality of the disabled I would urge a national policy of full employment. Clearly such a policy would not prevent disability but it could surely add to the opportunities available to most disabled persons to pay their own way, to socialize, and to regain and maintain their self-esteem. And it would enable many of the elderly to keep their jobs which would be the best bulwark against their focusing on the increasing aches and pains that tend to be by-products of aging.

Physicians and other health workers can do much more to address constructively the problems of the disabled and the chronically ill but the greatest contribution can be made by an enlightened public that deepens its understanding of the issues and prods its political representatives to institute preventive and remedial policies.

16

Care of the Dying: Two Vignettes

The three short pieces that follow address a single theme—the role of medicine in the care of the dying. This is a subject that most physicians prefer to avoid in a world in which malpractice suits and district attorneys in search of notoriety are ever-present threats. But the public keeps raising the issue anew, and it will not go away until we develop more understanding of what the choices are and how to assess them: the preferred procedures that should be followed to (1) allow optimal discretion for the competent individual to be involved in decisions affecting himself or herself; (2) to assure that legal surrogates can act on behalf of the noncompetent; and (3) to provide scope for professional judgment without giving physicians too much discretion in matters of life and death.

MY MOTHER

My mother reached her 93rd birthday in excellent health. Some arthritis and poor circulation in her legs bothered her but interfered neither with her living alone nor with her continuing her active life as volunteer, swimmer, fisherwoman, and world traveler. In the first half of her last year—she died one day before she would have been 94—she developed a condition that was diagnosed as sciatica, which caused her a great deal of pain and for which she received no effective therapy. But she was still able to manage on her own.

This account, however, concerns the last six months when her physical condition rapidly deteriorated and during which time she required full-time care at home and was hospitalized twice.

This is an abridged version of three articles originally titled "The High Costs of Dying," *Inquiry* 17:4 (293–95), Winter 1980; "More Care Is Not Always Better Care," *Inquiry* 19:3 (187–89), Fall 1982; and "The Elderly Are At Risk," *Inquiry* 21:4 (301–02), Winter 1984. Reprinted by permission.

My mother was fortunate in having the care of a local practitioner who specialized in geriatrics and also made house calls. In early December, after her physician had persuaded a senior cardiologist on the staff of St. Luke's Medical Center in New York City to see her at home, the decision was made to hospitalize her. Her breathing had become increasingly difficult, and at St. Luke's a diagnosis was made of congestive heart failure. After one lung was drained and she was placed on a regimen of standard drugs and medication to slow the rate of blood circulation, she did well. Her physician agreed with my preference to follow a plan of minimum intervention: to relieve her symptoms and to refrain from diagnostic explorations.

In the weeks prior to her first hospitalization, her physician put us in contact with several recent immigrants from Honduras who specialized in caring for geriatric patients. We needed coverage for weekdays, nights, and weekends. The cost per week came to around $600. When my mother was admitted to St. Luke's we brought these attendants with us, since it was immediately clear that the floor nursing was not adequate to provide the care she needed. A cot was rolled into her ample room for the night attendant. The hospital bill for her three weeks' stay came to just under $8,000. The physicians' fees were approximately $2,000. I was interested to observe the differences among physicians. Most did not accept assignment of their fees, and the one who did received about one-third of his fee from Medicare.

I have no way of knowing whether, or to what extent, the Hondurans were in the U.S. legally or illegally, but I do know they formed a closely knit group that threatened one of the peripheral members when, after my mother's return from the hospital, she agreed to work at a weekly rate considerably below that of the others. They threatened her and sought to bribe her with a better job, but since the job with my mother was a step up from her previous position she did not respond to their pressures. Her weekend relief was a Seventh Day Adventist from Jamaica, who had been trained as a nurse in Great Britain and who was studying for her R.N. examination in the States. The new cost for round-the-clock attendants amounted to about $350 weekly—a sizable reduction from the previous figure of $600.

Shortly after my mother returned home in early January she began to complain of intestinal pains, which diminished her desire for food and drink. When the pain worsened in early March she was forced to return to the hospital. Her physician had hoped to have her diagnosed as an outpatient, but she had weakened to a point where that was no longer practical. Without a clear-cut diagnosis, the attending gastroenterologist decided that she might be suffering from diverticulitis and began antibiotic treatment, which soon proved effective.

Once again she was released from the hospital after a three-week stay. This time, her hospital bill was slightly over $7,000, and the physicians' fees came to another $1,700. As during her first hospitalization, the two geriatric care attendants who cared for her at home continued to care for her during her hospital stay.

By now, her eyesight and hearing had weakened perceptibly, and after her second hospitalization my mother was even more disturbed by her increasing difficulties in walking. As long as she believed she was making progress, however slight, from one day to the next, her spirits held up. But by early April she began to question whether she had started on a permanent decline. At that point, she stopped making special efforts and began to sleep during much of each day.

Her last week was a nightmare because she developed acute pains, which pointed to kidney stones. When codeine failed to relieve the pain, she refused all food, liquid, and medication. I finally convinced her physician that we must move to another analgesic, and Demerol was selected. It is exceedingly difficult, however, to find druggists in Manhattan who will honor a legal prescription for a narcotic. Only repeated efforts yielded the amount she required, and on the third day after the Demerol injections were started, she died quietly in her sleep.

The total expenditures for the last six months of my mother's life are summarized as follows:

Physicians' fees	$ 5,000
Hospitalization—2 admissions	15,000
Round-the-clock geriatric care	10,000
Ambulance, drugs, laboratory tests, and sundries	1,000
	$31,000

Insurance covered a little more than half of these expenses.

A few questions, which have no easy answers, come to mind:

- How do families with limited resources cope with such costs of dying?
- If my mother's attending physician had been so inclined and if I had not discouraged him, it would have been easy to spend another $10,000 or more on diagnostic procedures during each hospitalization.
- My mother was close to death during her first hospitalization. All life-sustaining supports had been removed. Suppose she had not rallied? Money aside, was the pain she suffered thereafter compensated for by the prolongation of her life? No one had the right to prevent her rallying, but suppose we discover that most elderly people survive one or more painful episodes only to face increased suffering? What then?

THE ELDERLY AND ACCESS TO CARE

During the past few decades, the United States has broadened and deepened the access of the elderly and the poor to medical services. The recent White House Conference on Aging (December 1981) passed a series of recommendations that aimed at further improving medical services for the elderly.

Because of the shortages of operating and capital funds, the British have had to place constraints on the scope and depth of care that its National Health Service provides. In England, the elderly are ineligible in some instances for expensive diagnostic and therapeutic interventions; in other instances, patients go on waiting lists for nonemergency surgery and are treated in turn. Death frequently intervenes before the surgery is performed. In still other instances, patients obtain care on the private market, paying for the hospital bed and the physician out of their own pockets.

Health analysts have pointed out that differential access to care in the United States and the United Kingdom is not reflected in differences in longevity. The elderly die at approximately the same age whether or not they have had broad or limited access to sophisticated medical care. But as the late Walsh McDermott pointed out, longevity is not the appropriate criterion; reduced morbidity, greater ability to function, and reduction of pain and discomfort are the relevant measures.

The thrust of this brief discussion is to explore the facet of the current U.S. medical scene in which, because of Medicare, major medical, supplemental, and Medicaid coverage, the elderly have broad access to the most sophisticated care. Most of the economic barriers that in the past placed constraints on the access of the elderly to care have been removed. In addition, other factors encourage high utilization of sophisticated interventions. As in most other developed Western nations, religion, ethics, law, and medical tradition in the United States reinforce each other to create the consensus that the prolongation of life is an overriding national value. But the end of life is death, and no matter what we do, it can be postponed only briefly. As noted below, the efforts at postponement can lead to losses for the individual, the individual's family, and society.

The economic costs of heroic medical interventions late in the life of a patient are not my principal concerns, although a society such as ours, which spends much more on its elderly than on its young, may want to reconsider its allocations. In 1981, persons over 65, constituting about 11 percent of the total population, consumed about 30 percent of all health care expenditures; this came to roughly $2,635 per older person, in contrast to $370 for those under 19.[1] Again, my concern is less with economic considerations than with the McDermott criteria of reduced morbidity, greater ability to function, and reduction of pain and discomfort—which are more directly related to the quality of life.

Although some of the elderly are fully functioning one minute and dead the next as the result of a massive coronary attack or cerebral hemorrhage, most who reach their seventies or eighties exit more slowly. They are likely to suffer from one or more chronic diseases that slowly drain their strength and resistance until one of their critical systems is undermined. At that point, decision-making as to medical intervention becomes difficult. There are many diagnostic and therapeutic interventions that might be pursued, but many of them carry risks. Furthermore, the outlook for stabilization, amelioration, or cure of the ailing patient is reduced by the toll that has already taken place.

We need to rethink the role of medical intervention for most of the sick aged (as well as for others whose prognosis is poor) because of our ingrained tradition that looks upon the prolonging of life as a social imperative. Three factors are critical: the values of the patient, the medical decision-making process, and the risk/outcome ratio.

With respect to the patient's value system, we must realize that people feel differently about the prolongation of their lives. Some place a high value on extending their days, even if they will be confined to bed and suffer pain. Others see no point to living unless they can function as previously, able to carry on their work. Many fall in between. Since body and spirit are indissolubly linked, it is critically important that the patient's values and goals be factored into every medical decision, for it is the patient's future that is at stake.

Medicine today is specialized, which means that many decisions are made by consultants who do not know the patient as a person and who often do not have adequate knowledge of his or her medical history. Moreover, since most heroic interventions involve surgery and surgeons rarely carry responsibility for patient care beyond the walls of the operating room, their criterion of success is whether the patient survives the operation. They are less concerned with the patient's subsequent function or dysfunction. As one distinguished internist remarked recently, "After surgeons have done their jobs, they pass the old people back to us." They are not involved in the aftercare, in the patient's ability to function, in the quality of life that the patient faces.

We need a more explicit calculation of the risks and outcomes incident to the decision to operate or to otherwise resort to invasive technology in the care of the feeble elderly. The formulation that the patient will either survive the operation and walk out of the hospital cured or will die on the operating table is overly simplistic. There are many intervening outcomes, most of them bad. The patient may not die immediately but only after weeks or even months during which he or she endures a great amount of pain without hope or expectation of cure. The consequence of heroic interventions can be even more dysfunctional: a life of invalidism and dependency, sometimes including the loss of mental competence, extending over a period of years.

MY COUSIN

The foregoing principles were recently demonstrated in the terminal illness of a favorite cousin of mine. She was close to 78 and her job was the center of her life. She had no interest in continuing to live unless she could continue her work. Her recent medical history included several bouts of pneumonia, poor pulmonary function, and possible emphysema. The onset of her last illness was ushered in by severe weight loss. Unlike the earlier episodes, her physicians could not stabilize or reverse her illness. In desperation they decided upon cardiac catheterization. When the findings pointed to imminent closure of major vessels, they encouraged her to undergo, and pressed the cardiac surgeon to undertake, a quadruple bypass. The patient's decision was made easier by her knowledge that in the absence of surgery she was doomed to a life of semi-invalidism. The patient was told that the operation carried high risk, but she was also told that if she survived she could walk out cured and look forward to many good years of a fully functioning life. The surgery did not turn out as planned.

She did not die during the operation. Rather, she survived for five weeks, during which she suffered cardiac arrest, had to undergo a tracheotomy, was not lucid most of he time, could not be weaned from the oxygen flow, and, on the afternoon she died, was severely pummeled to enable her to breathe. It was clear at the end of the first postoperative week that she would not make it. Query: Assuming that the decision to operate was reasonable, should not a second decision have been made at this point to accept the new reality and treat her accordingly?

There must be ways to improve medical decision-making in a period that the language of the law describes as "in contemplation of death." Hippocrates addressed this critical issue: The physician must abstain from intentional harm. Physicians can avoid doing harm once they acknowledge that many elderly are beyond the stage where even modern medicine can help.

THE ELDERLY ARE AT RISK

There is growing disquietude that the elderly are at risk. Although Medicare covers less than half of their expenditures for health services, many experts are recommending larger deductibles and higher copayments in order to avoid the imminent deficit in the Trust Fund. Except for favoring a surcharge on Supplemental Medical Insurance premiums for those beneficiaries who pay income tax, I oppose the approach that would solve Medicare's fiscal problems by raising revenues from the elderly (See Chapter 17).

This analysis is concerned, however, less with financial risk and more with the dangers threatening the aged from "overtreatment" in acute care hospitals. Physicians, patients, and administrators recognize that third parties will in most instances cover the costs of whatever treatment plan is selected. As the competition for patients intensifies, acute care hospitals face increasing pressure to keep their beds filled, with the paradoxical result that the sick elderly are in jeopardy.

Recent advances in medicine, in particular improved surgical technique and supportive care, have encouraged physicians to pursue ever bolder treatment plans. Until the last decade or two, few of the very old were evaluated for surgery and even fewer were operated upon. Today the factor of age, per se, is no longer considered in the choice of a treatment plan that may include surgery for a ninety-year old.

There are unquestionably tens of thousands of elderly persons both in and out of nursing homes for whom medical evaluation and care in an acute hospital are indicated. Many could profit from surgery which would add to their functionality and well-being. This note calls attention to the tens of thousands of other aged individuals who find themselves in an acute hospital where they and their physician must decide whether to proceed with a more or less radical plan of treatment.

Most patients and most physicians, especially residents, are so convinced of the curative powers of modern medicine, that they all but deny the inevitability of death. Small wonder, therefore, that more and more patients in their late eighties and even nineties are being operated upon; that many are maintained by life-sustaining supports; and that still others undergo debilitating chemotherapy.

The foregoing observations are not intended to deny the sick elderly access to the armamentarium of modern medicine, the way our poor English cousins have been forced by budgetary constraints,[2] but rather to raise the issue whether unlimited access may not prove dysfunctional for many.

As individuals approach the end of their lives, their physical reserves are far depleted, and this depletion militates against the success of complex medical procedures. Under these conditions, the preferred way to deal with terminal illness is to resort to narcotics for the relief of pain and permit the patient gradual release into oblivion and death, sparing him the agony and indignity of a struggle he cannot win.

Our increasingly sophisticated health care system needs to reassess the potential and limitations of radical interventions in the case of the sick elderly. Both patients and physicians must appraise the facts realistically and the one element that must never be left out of the equation is the narrowing gap between advancing age and certain death that leaves less and less room for therapeutic medicine.

The judgments that must be made are difficult enough without being complicated by the fact that many hospitals have an economic stake in doing more for the dying patient. There are many reasons for removing excess beds from the system, but none more persuasive than the importance of protecting the sick elderly from the dangers of overtreatment.

17

The Reform of Medicare: A Plea for Caution

As with every issue on its agenda, Congress can consider the reform of Medicare from a narrow or a broad perspective and can respond through modest or far-reaching action.

In addition to the obvious fact that Medicare will face a financial crisis in the years ahead, it has other serious shortcomings: it does not provide insurance for catastrophic illness; long-term care, a major need of the frail and sick elderly, is not covered; the proportion of the health care costs of the elderly that Medicare covers has declined since the beginning of the program to a point where it accounts for less than half of their total outlays for medical care. About two-thirds of all Medicare beneficiaries buy Medigap insurance to protect themselves against the high deductible items and other forms of cost-sharing mandated by Medicare. Medigap, which has a high loading cost, probably contributes to the over-use of scarce resources by discouraging patients and their physicians from pursuing less costly but efficacious forms of treatment. And until the recent introductions of TEFRA and DRG, Medicare's reimbursement policies surely contributed to steep acceleration of hospital costs.

In light of the foregoing catena of shortcomings, the approaching financial crisis might be viewed by Congress as an opportunity to undertake a radical restructuring not only of Medicare but of our total health care system. I am convinced that such an effort would be misguided and would surely fail.

Let me briefly explain why I have reached this conclusion and why I believe that Congress would be well advised to focus largely, perhaps exclusively, on the one problem that it must address, the prospective large

Originally published in Subcommittee on Health, Committee on Ways and Means, U.S. House of Representatives, *Proceedings of the Conference on the Future of Medicare* (Washington D.C.: GPO, 1984), pp. 49–54.

deficit in the Medicare Trust Fund, at the same time that it seeks to reduce general fund support for Supplemental Medical Insurance. The following brief review is a reminder of earlier efforts to improve and reform Medicare.

Since 1972, there have been repeated federal legislative and administrative actions aimed at slowing the rise in hospital costs, the key element in Medicare expenditures, accounting for about 70 percent of its total outlays. There is only one way to read this record. We have had little success in containing the rise in costs. The most that can be said for more than a decade's efforts is that, without them, the increases would have been still greater. We are just starting on a new, much more radical, effort, the DRG approach. The better part of wisdom would be to give this initiative a chance to show what it can do. DRG may not work and it surely won't work without adjustments down the road as the full import and impact of prospective care reimbursement are revealed. But if Congress, in responding to the looming financial crisis facing Medicare, were to introduce additional changes, it would almost certainly doom the DRG system before it has a chance to demonstrate its potential for reducing the rate of hospital cost increases.

It is a decade since Congress decided to make federal funding available to accelerate the growth of HMOs in the hope and expectation that they would be able to contain health care costs. However, the rules and regulations were drawn so tight that growth was inhibited; even after the regulations were relaxed, HMOs have grown relatively slowly and with regard to enrolling Medicare beneficiaries on a prepayment basis, the record of the HMOs to date is close to nil. HMOs are simply not able or willing to risk adverse selection.

During the last decade, there has been a proliferation of alternative health care delivery systems and the years ahead will see many more but it would be an error to exaggerate the speed with which the extant system of fee-for-service medicine, private sector Blue Cross-Blue Shield and commercial insurance, the increasing technological sophistication of nonprofit acute hospitals, and the academic health centers are changing or will change.

More than six years ago Alain Enthoven first recommended to the Secretary of HEW that the basic structure of the U.S. medical care system be altered through greater reliance on the "competitive market." His was the most far-reaching proposal advanced to change the existing incentives which determine the behavior of both consumers and providers. He hoped to accomplish the following: to improve efficiency through more appropriate treatment modalities, assure broad access to health care for the poor, to reduce federal outlays, provide insurance for catastrophic illness, and much more. All of these benefits, he maintained, would be obtained at a considerably reduced total cost. His cogently written proposal had one major flaw: he did not explain how or why the key interest groups—physicians, academic health centers, trade union members, and the elderly—should embrace "competition" if their losses were certain, their gain problematic.

The foregoing abbreviated account suggests that it is much easier for analysts to outline on paper the design of a much improved health care system than for Congress to legislate the reforms to affect it. It is just possible that the extant Medicare system, while far from perfect, has been performing reasonably well, which is all that one can expect in this imperfect world. It has brought the elderly into the mainstream of American medicine. Their access to health care has been much expanded. They are reasonably protected against high bills for acute hospitalization. They are being treated by physicians who, because of advances in knowledge and technology, can do more for them by adding to both the quality of their lives and their longevity.

Since the expenditures of the Medicare program have risen much more rapidly than anticipated and the total costs for health care are now at 10.5 percent of GNP and continuing to rise, the federal government must shore up the Medicare Trust Fund. This is the principal challenge that Congress confronts. The public is not asking Congress to alter in any radical fashion the Medicare system as it has evolved; it is even less interested in restructuring the entire health care system. Although many are concerned about the steeply rising health care costs, there is no political consensus for major Medicare or total health care reform.

THE HSAIO-KELLY PROPOSAL

In light of my reading of our experience with Medicare, I will now comment briefly on Professor William Hsaio's and Ms. Nancy L. Kelly's paper "Restructuring Medicare Benefits." I will also add some recommendations for Congress to consider in its forthcoming review of and response to Medicare's approaching financial crisis. The Hsaio-Kelly paper is at once too ambitious and not ambitious enough. It deals with possible ways of helping to close the financial gap that looms ahead but its recommendations go only a small distance in this direction—a $3 billion contribution towards closing the gap by 1987. At the same time the authors recommend the introduction of a major new benefit—"catastrophic coverage." Further, they contend that their detailed proposals, if implemented, would lead to desirable changes in the actions of both beneficiaries and providers which would contribute to the more efficient use of health care resources which in turn would be reflected in lower costs.

It seems to me to be counter-indicated to recommend any new costly benefit such as catastrophic coverage at a time when the prospective Trust

Fund deficit may approach or exceed $300 billion by 1995. The issue of catastrophic insurance has been on and off the congressional agenda for many years but even when the financial situation of Medicare and the federal government was much more favorable than at present, the key committees declined to mark up a bill. If they had reasons to hesitate in the late 1970s, they have much better reasons to delay in the mid-1980s. I agree with the authors that in theory any broad insurance plan should include catastrophic coverage. For better or worse, however, the American public has defined medical insurance as a system of protection not against financial ruin but rather freedom from having to pay out-of-pocket for large medical bills. Since the public has repeatedly demonstrated that it is not willing to copay more, to add coverage for catastrophic illness appears at this time to be ill advised.

Moreover, I question the emphasis which the authors place upon those facets of their proposal aimed at changing the behavior of both consumers and providers. If one starts with the premise that most Americans have an ongoing relationship with a physician whom they trust and whose advice they generally follow and further that they have coverage that protects them against large bills, there is little room for incentives based on price to come into play. Similarly, while long-term changes in the number of physicians can affect their fee schedules and how they practice, the established members of the profession have considerable scope at present and in the near and middle term to continue more or less in their accustomed ways. Over time the new entrants into the profession will have to adjust to a more crowded market and will be under pressure to join an alternative delivery system or accept salaried positions. But one must not assume that if these shifts occur total costs will be constrained. I doubt it.

With regard to hospital care, patients follow their physicians' advice both as to admission and treatment. The DRG system looks to price competition to slow costs but whether it will succeed remains to be seen. Finally, alternative delivery systems focused on price will have some effect on the present system but it will be slow. I would give relatively little weight to the authors' anticipation of major efficiency gains; prices alone cannot alter fundamentally a market in which consumers pay out-of-pocket only about 30 percent of all charges and in the case of hospital care, less than 10 percent. Since most consumers have broad insurance coverage and since physicians are wedded to fee-for-service, price competition will not bring about significant efficiency gains. Only a radical restructuring of the entire system, such as Enthoven envisaged, which neither a Democratic nor Republican administration was willing to try, could provide the market test which the authors favor.

I do not believe that Congress should attempt to modify the Medicare system by placing a sizable copayment on most patients who use hospitals between the 2nd and 60th day. That would be a major "take-back" from the elderly, half of whom have very modest incomes, no more than twice the poverty level.

My primary objections to the authors' proposal therefore are fourfold: it provides too little relief for the financial situation facing Medicare; it offers a new and costly benefit, that for catastrophic illness; it suggests, mistakenly in my opinion, that there will be large efficiency gains that will moderate the rise in costs; it ignores the violation of the "social contract" by reducing substantially the benefits that Medicare has provided beneficiaries up to the present.

I have a series of second-order objections which I will briefly note. I see no way of establishing and operating a threefold classification system of providers, physicians, and hospitals, based on their relative charges, and gearing copayments accordingly. The administrative and legal complications of shifting classifications in a rapidly changing marketplace would be horrendous and the realignments in patient-physician and physician-hospital relations would either not occur or if they did the ensuing costs would be very large. I consider it bad public policy to encourage patients to seek medical care according to unit price; the much more relevant considerations should be safety and long-term efficacy.

Further the authors slip when they provide a figure of $120 as the average additional cost per beneficiary. Only one in five of the elderly is hospitalized in any one year and there is a high probability that those admitted will have a second hospitalization during the following year. Accordingly the potential costs should be calculated not in terms of all beneficiaries but for those who require hospitalization. The costs to the latter would be many times the average figure for all beneficiaries.

Finally the authors assume that the preference for Medigap policies would be reduced by the expansion of Medicare coverage under their proposal to include protection against catastrophic costs. From what we have said earlier, I doubt that many beneficiaries would forego this protection. In that event, the so-called behavioral changes aimed at cost containment on the part of providers would be problematic.

I believe that the major contribution of the Hsaio-Kelly proposal is to alert the Congress to move with great circumspection before it decides to legislate any broad-based reforms for Medicare.

A FEW MODEST SUGGESTIONS

Congress should focus its attention on finding new sources of income for the Trust Fund. My own preferences are for increasing the tax rate on HI, introducing a premium geared to income for beneficiary payments for SMI, and increasing revenues through higher excise taxes on cigarettes, liquor, and known carcinogenic substances. In addition, Congress should explore whether the following might over time make a lesser or greater contribution to slowing the rate of increase of health care costs without depriving beneficiaries of significant current benefits.

HMOs should be encouraged to accept Medicare enrollees on a prepayment basis by enabling them to protect themselves against adverse selection factors through higher premiums based on the health status of potential enrollees. There is no need in my opinion to complicate this issue by tying it to a voluntary, and surely not to a mandatory, voucher system.

Since there is widespread agreement among knowledgeable persons that the rapid and continuing introduction of new technology has been a major contributor to a steady and steep rise in health care costs, an advisory commission under professional leadership might help to slow the acceptance of new costly procedures until they have demonstrated significant therapeutic value.

An early effort should be made to provide an alternative to the present pass-through of capital costs under the DRG system aimed at containing, and reducing, the nation's acute bed capacity.

Too little is known about the 1 percent of all patients who account for 30 percent of all medical expenditures, up from 17 percent in the period just before the passage of Medicare and Medicaid. The presumption is that if we understood the reasons back of these very large expenditures, some alternative, less costly therapeutic approaches might be used.

One concluding comment: I do not believe that all of the foregoing, even if aggressively pursued, will prevent health care costs from continuing to increase as a percentage of GNP. But to interdict such a rise is not the challenge that Congress faces nor is it one that Congress has the capacity to resolve. The federal government accounts for over one-quarter of all health care expenditures, a significant proportion but not enough to leverage the system. At some point down the road the other major participants may become so unnerved by the continuing rise in total health care expenditures that they may seek new federal legislation aimed at restructuring the system. At that point Congress will be better positioned to act. Until that time, it should find a solution for the difficult but much less complex issue of keeping Medicare financially viable.

18

The Coming Struggle for the Health Care Dollar

There are only three significant sources of funds for health care: government, which accounts for over 40 percent of all health care dollars; insurance, which provides just under 30 percent; and the consumer's pocket, which provides the remaining 30 percent. Over 40 percent of the total goes to hospitals, if we include both inpatient and outpatient services. Since nursing homes take almost another 10 percent, institutional care consumes about one-half of all health care dollars. While physicians are very important in the running of the system, they do not walk home, as many people believe, with all the money. They receive fewer than one of five of the dollars that flow into the system.

Everything else—dentists, laboratories, insurance premiums, and the administration of the health insurances system—is paid for with the remaining 30 percent.

Let's review the winners and the losers in the struggle for the health care dollar over the last twenty years. Since the inception of Medicare and Medicaid in 1965, the acute care hospitals, particularly the larger sophisticated institutions, have received a larger share of a much larger total. Suburban hospitals have also been winners, because we have almost duplicated our hospital plant. We used to have hospitals primarily in cities and in sizable communities. Now there is also a major system of suburban hospitals.

Nursing homes have been the third big winner. There may not be enough of them and they may not be of the quality we would like, but since shortly before Medicare and Medicaid were established, nursing homes have grown from roughly 1 percent to 10 percent of the system's revenues.

Originally published in *Critical Issues in Health Care Management,* Issue 2, The Mount Sinai School of Medicine, New York, 1983, pp. 15–16. Reprinted by permission.

According to the American Medical Association, physicians have not been faring so well recently but that is a misconception. The individual physician has had to cope with inflation just like the rest of the population. However, doctors have maintained their relative position despite a substantial increase in physician manpower. While physician incomes did not improve in the 1970s, neither did they go down. Physicians actually did pretty well in the face of a rapidly expanding supply.

Among the subgroups of physicians who made major gains are the house staffs, who used to earn a pittance before Medicare and Medicaid, and foreign medical graduates. Because we did not expand our medical schools in the United States until almost the 1970s, there was a lot of room in the system for foreigners to establish themselves successfully in the practice of medicine in this country. Today about one-quarter of all practicing physicians in the United States are graduates of foreign medical schools.

These were the big winners in a period of flush money. Who were the losers? Public hospitals. Think, for example, of what has happened to our state mental institutions. They followed the so-called logic of emptying their patients into the street, but in my opinion such action had more to do with budgets than with logic. Look at Philadelphia Hospital, Cook County Hospital in Chicago, and Kings County Hospital in Brooklyn: these public hospitals were hit hard. Public health departments also were losers. And in a perverse way, the so-called cutting edge of the new delivery systems was a loser. Take HMOs. California has several, Washington D.C. and New York City each had one, but they really did not take off. The community health centers that the federal government financed under various programs also were losers because they never became an integral part of the delivery system.

Specific groups of physicians also lost, particularly psychiatrists and pediatricians. And, in a period when new money was pouring into the system, all nonphysicians, including nurses and technicians, did relatively poorly, despite the fact that the health sector experienced a tremendous increase in total employment.

Now that the stage is set, I shall explain why the struggle for the health care dollar is going to heat up. First, bear in mind that government is the single largest source of money for health care: it contributes about 42 percent of all dollars with the federal government providing almost a third of the total. And the federal government now has the worst deficit in its history, with even greater deficits looming in the future, the like of which no economist could have even imagined a few years ago. The Congressional Budget Office estimates deficits of $1.1 to $1.5 trillion within the next five years. I was in Germany in 1922, so I have seen a country that devalued its currency until there was nothing left. I do not think we are going to do the same in this country. The only choice we have is to exercise control over the federal budget.

State and local governments—primarily state governments—also have a stake in this struggle. Even poor states must contribute a considerable amount of Medicaid money, and state budgets these days are very constrained. In New York, 50 percent of all Medicaid money comes from state and local governments and the State of New York is facing a budget deficit of between $1.6 and $1.9 billion. This gap has to be closed because New York is not able, like to the federal government, to print money.

In some states, including North Carolina and Maryland, Medicaid pays for up to fourteen days of hospitalization for a medically indigent patient. If the patient is still hospitalized on the fifteenth day, the hospital has to cover the costs in some way. A large number of states have already tightened admissions to nursing homes and many poor people have been taken off the Medicaid rolls. We are experiencing an actual diminution of services and, in my opinion, this is only the beginning of our budget troubles.

There is a third party involved in the financing of health care. Almost 30 percent of the money that flows into the health care system comes from insurance. The bulk of this money originates in the collective bargaining agreements between workers and employers. Some of the resulting costs are astronomical; for example, in the current United Automotive Workers contract which covers both active and laid-off workers and retirees, the cost of health insurance to the employer is about $5,000 annually per employed worker. Health insurance costs automotive employers more than steel, their basic raw material. It is not surprising, therefore, that business and labor coalitions are saying to Blue Cross and commercial insurers, "We cannot afford continuing increases in premiums. You must do more to control costs."

Another particularly important factor is that the production of physicians is out of control. In the short run this cannot be mitigated because new doctors are already in the pipeline. But look at the facts. In 1950, there were about 140 physicians per 100,000 population, and people were not dropping dead because of medical neglect. Now we have over 200 physicians for every 100,000 people. This is a substantial increase, but it occurred slowly over the thirty-year period of 1950–80. But from 1980 to 1990 the number of physicians per 100,000 people will rise to 240, and the best government figures suggest that we shall be up to 280 by the end of the century.

While physicians, as we have seen, do not take home all or even most of the bacon, they do have a tremendous influence on how much money is spent. The greater the surplus of physicians, the greater the likelihood that health care costs will go up. Even when there is no financial incentive, professional people prefer to keep busy—you can imagine what will happen if they have to keep busy in order to make a living.

Another significant event is that the health care industry stopped expanding in the early to mid-1970s, not in terms of dollars but in terms of services: both inpatient care days and ambulatory visits are declining. We are seeing the end of a period in which the American public was enamored with medicine. Since the end of World War II, medicine has been able to offer a great deal. But now people have learned that you might pick up an infection in a hospital and that occasionally anesthesia equipment does not work. The public has become somewhat less enamored of and less trusting about what medicine can do.

Until now, the hospital has been a wonderful workplace for physicians. It allowed them to optimize time by seeing more patients and using the services of the house staff. But as dollars become progressively scarcer, some physicians are making diagnostic and therapeutic work in their own offices or at group clinics. This phenomenon, known as "unbundling" of ancillary services, will present many hospitals with serious financial losses.

Another factor is that a number of well capitalized profit-making institutions are in a good position to pick off a lucrative part of the market and in the process make lots of money. According to *Medical Economics,* within the next few years Humana expects to invest $1 billion in emergency centers. These centers will directly compete with fee-for-service private practitioners. We will see more such efforts by profit-making medicine to find an expanded place in the market.

To sum up: the federal and state budgets and the insurance system are under pressure; an extraordinarily large number of physicians will soon be competing with each other to make a living; and the competitive environment will increase as the profit-making sector vies with the nonprofit sector for the available dollars.

What do I think the first order consequences will be? It is inevitable, and this is one of the few forecasts I am sure about, that physicians' incomes will decline substantially. This does not mean that the best-established surgeons or other specialists will be affected. It does mean that young people entering the profession will have considerably fewer earning capabilities than expected. But there is no sacred rule that, after practicing for three years upon completion of their residency, physicians are entitled to make $100,000 or more. I do not plan to worry about the fact that they will probably earn a lower income. I have never been a great believer in public policies directed at reducing physicians' incomes, but it is going to happen.

I also expect that physicians will soon lean on state legislatures to cut back medical school enrollment. I also think there will be at least partial success in reducing the inflow of not only foreign medical graduates, but also of U.S. citizens who are graduates of foreign medical schools.

Delivery mechanisms such as HMOs, emergency centers, and hospitals that hire salaried physicians will have a much easier time. The reason HMOs have grown slowly was that they did not appeal to physicians. Now HMOs will be more attractive because an increasing number of young doctors will have difficulties getting established. As proof for this, I talked some time ago with the chief physician at Kaiser Permanente who told me that he was able to hire physicians at the same salary offered the year before and at the same time attracted quality applicants.

We are going to see more corporate medicine of all sorts, including hospital medicine. Some of the more aggressive hospitals will hire full-time staff because doctors will be willing to work for a reasonable salary. And I expect to see all kinds of deal-making among hospitals, outlying satellite clinics, HMOs, and the like, because patients will be scarce and providers will compete for them. Patients are already fairly scarce. The U.S. hospital system operates at around 70 percent capacity. While some hospitals are full, and some may even be overflowing, on the whole we have too many beds.

I expect to see new competition between hospitals and physicians. The best chance for physicians to maintain their income will be to reduce to the minimum the number of patients they send to the hospital. The hospitals, in turn, will be very interested in having more patients admitted. I think a considerable number of hospitals will become quite aggressive in providing primary care in the community, putting group practices together in outpatient departments and in the emergency rooms. This is happening now in the public health care system in New York City.

Whoever can control the flow of patients will have an asset of considerable value because patients, as mentioned earlier, are going to be scarce, especially insured patients. We can expect more unbundling of services that currently provide hospitals, especially major hospitals, with a large part of their revenues. Many of these services, including much minor surgery, will be performed outside the hospital.

Physicians have always been reluctant to hand over their functions to other health practitioners and this attitude is going to harden. In a period of worsening economics, there is nothing that a physician now controls which he will be willing to let go.

There will be tighter reimbursement systems, and hospitals will be looking very carefully at whom they admit, how they treat them, and whom they refer. Referrals from one hospital to another are already much restricted, except for those patients a hospital does not want.

One response of hospitals to tightening reimbursements and leveling off of referrals will be diversification. Some will deliver different types of ambulatory care, some will link up with nursing homes, and others will provide home health care. These will provide ways to extend the hospital. I look forward to some gains in quality from some of these developments. And I expect to see a substantial reduction in the number of freestanding small hospitals. They will face increasing difficulties because these hospitals are poorly positioned to purchase economically, make use of new technology, and gain access to the capital market without which they will find it difficult to survive.

Borrowing capital is going to be more difficult because hospitals in the past financed themselves through debt based on the reimbursement system. Once that becomes problematic, as in Massachusetts where the amount of reimbursement will go down each year for the next three years under their waiver system, Wall Street will take another view of the matter. Hospitals will not be able to borrow so easily under the new reimbursement systems that are being put in place.

So much for first order consequences; now let us look at the second order consequences.

First, it was nonsense to broadcast that the United States would establish a single standard of health care for the American people. That was a fantasy, not a social goal. That must be clear by now.

Second, the real danger is that some people, the poor and especially the near-poor, are without health insurance. Our basic health insurance is tied to employment and we had recently ten and a half million unemployed people. According to the President's own forecast, we are going to remain at a relatively high level of unemployment for the next three or four years, which means that there will continue to be a large number of people without health insurance.

Third, most states will be looking for every possible way to get their health care costs under control. Just think of what California is in the process of doing: the hospital that presents the lowest bid gets the contract for Medicaid patients. The major university hospital in San Francisco suddenly found itself with 33 percent of its beds empty because it did not get a Medicaid contract. We can expect to see more and more disruption.

Fourth, the health industry is based on cross-subsidization. Healthy people who are lucky take care of the unlucky people who get sick. That is the only way to make the insurance system work. Moreover, hospitals always used cross-subsidization to balance their books. If Medicare did not pay all of its costs, hospitals put a little extra on commercial insurance or on the patients who paid their own bills. Hospitals can no longer do that in Massachusetts or in New York. This will place additional financial pressure on the more expensive institutions.

Under Medicare, elderly patients now pay for one day of hospitalization and the next 59 days cost them nothing. President Reagan proposes that they make a copayment from the second to the sixtieth day. Depending on length of hospitalization, that can represent to the elderly hundreds of thousands of dollars of copayments. I do not think the President will get his proposal passed, surely not the first time around, but that is what he is asking for. He is also asking to freeze for one year the fees of physicians who take care of Medicare patients.

I do not know where the proliferation of new delivery systems will take us. Some naive economists think new delivery systems will save us a lot of money. I believe it is possible that it will increase the total costs of the system. In the short and intermediate terms, if new ambulatory surgery facilities are built and hospital capacity is not reduced, we shall see only more outlays, not less.

In any one year, about 8 percent of Medicare patients use about 70 percent of all Medicare money. We know that most of these high cost patients are in their final year of life. Aside from the dollar question, I believe that we are doing too much to, not for, the dying patient. Again, aside from costs, I think it is bad medical practice. The moribund ought to be permitted to die quietly, free of pain, and with dignity.

This overtreatment of the elderly came about in part because physicians are trained to do everything possible for patients and in part because Americans believe in the prolongation of life. Add to this the specter of malpractice and we understand why we are spending so much money on older people. I believe that slowly we will get a little more sensible about how best to treat them. A first change has already occurred. Under the tax law revision of August 1982, dying patients can use some of their Medicare benefits for hospice rather than hospital care. In addition, the President is asking for an option which he will probably get that will allow the elderly to choose an HMO rather than Medicare.

I think we will see a lot more entrepreneurial medicine from health care providers, both profit-making and nonprofit, individual doctors, and hospitals. Whether this competition will reduce costs remains problematic; I do not pretend to know how it will work out.

Standard-setting will take on new significance. I think discrepancies in costs per episode for the same types of patients in different parts of the country will end, although this will not happen overnight. I do not think hospitals in New York City will have to match the national average length of stay, this year or next, but there is no question that we are going to make more use of statistical controls to moderate costs.

In conclusion, the struggle for the health care dollar can only intensify because we are going to have a reduced inflow of total dollars and a greater number of physicians at a time when the industry's demand is leveling off. There will be increased pressure on sophisticated hospitals because these hospitals are much more than service institutions: they are major educational and research organizations, and their additional costs up to now have been covered through reimbursement. If the reimbursement net develops bigger and bigger holes, as it will, I do not know how many of these major institutions are going to make it. Moreover, in the period of turmoil which I anticipate, there will be room for all kinds of entrepreneurs, many of whom will be phony but some of whom will be efficient. That is what usually happens in a new industry or when an old industry starts to change. The most dangerous aspect is what is going to happen to the poor and the near-poor who will be at increasing risk. It is inconceivable to let poor, sick people die without proper medical care, but the signs are ominous: in some high unemployment areas, infant mortality rates are up. It is clear that more trouble lies ahead. Unless we want to turn our backs on our tradition, commitment, and values, we must ask society to find the money to ensure that all persons, including all of the poor, continue to have access to medical care.

Afterword

The Power Shift

This concluding chapter will address the interactions between the elements of continuity that have shaped American medicine during the last third of a century and the elements of change which are emerging and which will reshape the system by the century's end. First, we will recall the significant changes which we have earlier identified: dollar outlays that increased from around $13 billion in 1950 to $362 billion in 1983; the expansion of the supply of physicians which resulted in a 50 percent increase in the ratio of physicians per 100,000 population, from 140 to 210; the change in the length of physician training, close to 100 percent, from five to ten years plus or minus and a shift from general practice to specialties and subspecialties; the increased scale and sophistication of the nation's hospitals, including a partial replication of the urban system in the suburbs and smaller communities; the explosive growth of health insurance from around a few billion dollars to over $80 billion and after 1965 the explosive growth in government payments for medical care for the elderly and the poor which together approached $100 billion in 1983; the expansion in new modes of physician practice including single specialty groups, multispecialty groups, preferred provider plans, salaried employment, and the continuation of many in solo arrangements; and finally the explosive growth in the numbers of other health professionals, nurses, and allied health workers.

The changes which have been identified above together with many others such as the approximate doubling in the number of U.S. medical schools, the large inflows of foreign-trained physicians, and the blossoming of biomedical research make it difficult, at least initially, to see the points of continuity in the health care sector. On first inspection it appears that all of the key parameters have been altered, most of them radically.

But a closer view reveals a significant number of important continuities during this tumultuous third of a century. Most Americans continue to obtain their routine (ambulatory) health care from a physician of their choice just as had been their practice in earlier generations. Most physicians continue to practice fee-for-service medicine which means that their patients pay their bills although a growing percentage of them are reimbursed in whole or in part by insurance, or, if they are older, by Medicare.

When patients become seriously ill they are admitted to a hospital for inpatient treatment, just as in earlier times. True, the diagnostic and therapeutic interventions which they undergo have become more sophisticated and many are cured of conditions for which earlier there had been no effective treatment. However, the financing of hospital care has been radically altered: Third parties, that is, insurance and government, now cover over 90 percent of all hospital bills.

The last paragraphs suggest that the element of continuity still dominates the manner in which patients receive medical care from their physicians at the same time that considerable change has occurred in the manner in which the care is paid for as a consequence of the major growth in private insurance and in the share of the costs carried by government. The government's share has increased from about 25 percent in 1950 to 42 percent today or closer to 50 percent if the value of tax expenditure benefits is added to direct public outlays.

The easiest way to summarize the relative influences of continuity and change in the American health care sector during the last third of the century is to realize, as we have just stated, that the practice of medicine has not been radically altered while the financing of the system has been substantially transformed. Since total dollar outlays for health have increased more than 27 times during this period, the health care sector has become 2–1/2 times greater as a share of a substantially enlarged GNP.

In a society such as ours in which the behavior of the individual as well as of the citizenry at large is affected by the availability of money, it is surprising to find such large alterations as have occurred in health care expenditures without antecedent, concomitant, or subsequent alterations in the values, power, and politics of the principal institutions that dominate the sector. Accordingly we must look more closely at the medical establishment, both its foundations and superstructure, to determine whether the element of continuity which appears to dominate in 1985 may mask cracks and fissures which, if evaluated and projected, would point to significant changes in the remaining years of this century. The title of this concluding chapter—The Power Shift—seeks to convey a double message: many shifts in the power constellation have already occurred, although they have not been fully appreciated and many more are imminent and will soon become manifest.

If we use 1950 as a point of departure to assess the extent to which the decision-making fulcrum in American medicine has shifted, we find that in the immediate postwar years, the medical profession, both the practitioner and the organized establishment, the American Medical Association, with its national, state, and county societies, dominated the health care sector and no group was interested in or able to challenge them. Although the trustees of nonprofit hospitals were responsible for raising the philanthropic funds that determined the number and sophistication of inpatient treatment facilities, they took their cues from their senior staff physicians who pressed for more beds and more modern equipment.

State legislatures had several discrete but delimited roles. They appropriated much of the funds required to finance medical education; they had the legal power to license physicians and other health providers, a task which they generally delegated to the respective professions, and they were responsible for caring for patients with chronic illness, particularly the large numbers of mental patients. They, and the localities over which they exercised jurisdiction, together shared the responsibility for a wide variety of public health measures.

The federal government played a modest role, responsible for providing medical care to members of the Armed Forces, selected groups of veterans, and for providing some care to special populations such as American Indians and merchant seamen.

To complete the roster we would have to take note of the role of nonprofit universities, several of which operated prestigious medical schools such as Harvard, Columbia, University of Pennsylvania, and Johns Hopkins; large, for-profit pharmaceutical firms; and a small proprietary hospital sector.

In contrast to other established professional groups, including the clergy, the military, academicians, lawyers, engineers—all of which were heavily dependent on other powerful groups, private, nonprofit, and government, for facilities and resources to realize their goals and objectives—physicians were able to practice medicine with only infrequent and modest interference from others. By law, tradition, and practice only physicians could treat the sick and injured. They were responsible to themselves, their peers, and their patients. The fact that they earned their livelihood from the fees they charged their patients reinforced their freedom and independence, especially in the immediate post-World War II era when the demand for their services outpaced their numbers.

It is not immediately clear why in a third of a century that saw so many favorable developments—the increased technological potential of modern medicine, the deepening of its knowledge base, the broadening of its service delivery, widespread public support which resulted in a great inflow of new resources—there was a significant decline in the power of physicians, a decline that is likely to accelerate in the remaining years of this century.

We can identify the following major forces that directly or indirectly altered the balance of power. There was a change in the attitude of the

American people towards medical care as a result of the exposure of 15 million servicemen and their dependents to the quality care which the War and Navy Departments provided. Although the United States has balked at putting in place a governmental system which would provide universal access to health care, it has moved toward that goal through a series of stages, using both governmental and nongovernmental institutions and resources. This change in values which has stopped just short of declaring health care as a right, brought government, both federal and state, from the periphery into the center of political decision-making. The first erosion of the power of physicians was directly and indirectly brought about by the realization of the public that physicians could not be relied upon to provide an acceptable level of care to the many millions who were unable to pay for their own care.

A second major change that helped to undermine the leadership and hegemony of organized medicine came from the emergence of the major biomedical research effort, financed overwhelmingly by the federal government. The billions of dollars that started to flow into the academic health centers created a new and distinctive constituency within the medical establishment, represented by the American Association of Medical Colleges and their allied groups whose leadership, while continuing to share interests and goals with the AMA, had its own agenda, an agenda which made it more receptive to an expanded role for the federal government. In 1950, the AMA shared with the Catholic Church unparalled influence in the halls of Congress when it came to deflecting legislative initiatives to which it objected. In 1985, the leaders of key committees feel free to mark up bills that the AMA opposes, with little concern that this will make them vulnerable at the next election. American medicine no longer speaks with a single voice.

In the years before the passage of Medicare and Medicaid federal outlays for all health care amounted to about $5 billion; in 1983 the total was more than $100 billion greater. The states, largely because of their partial financing of Medicaid, have also made substantially enlarged outlays for health. Despite President Reagan's expressed policy to expand spending for defense and to control outlays for domestic programs, federal appropriations for health are the most steeply rising item in the federal budget. When President Johnson traveled to President Truman's home in Independence, Missouri to sign the amendments to the Social Security Act that established Medicare and Medicaid he had no inkling that in a relatively short period of time it would become a wild card in the federal budget. This lack of prevision helps to explain why he was willing to assure the AMA that, in exchange for the organization's willingness to accommodate the new legislation, the federal government would eschew altering in any substantial manner the pattern of patient-physician relations which were grounded in fee-for-service medical care.

But Johnson's successors began a slow but steady retreat by putting into place in 1972 the Professional Standards Review Organization (PSRO), in 1973, federal subsidies for approved health maintenance organizations (HMOs), in 1974, health planning legislation, in 1976, new health manpower legislation aimed at affecting the proportion of generalists versus specialists and through related legislation affecting the distribution of physicians to encourage their practicing in underserved areas. In 1980 the Secretary of the Department of Health, Education, and Welfare released the results of the Graduate Medical Education National Advisory Committee which had spent four years estimating and assessing the outlook for physician and other health personnel for 1990 and 2000 and which concluded that a substantial "surplus" loomed ahead.

Within the short span of the last twenty years the federal government, which had been kept by the AMA at arm's length from playing a direct role in the shaping and reshaping of American medicine, has come to assume a dominant role in affecting directly the access of the elderly and the poor to health care services; the numbers, specialization, and location of many members of the profession; the emergence and growth of preferred systems of health care delivery to compete head-on with the profession's preference for fee-for-service arrangements; and in 1984 passing legislation that for the third time since 1971 placed a ceiling on all, or some part, of physicians' fees. Starting in October 1983, the federal government also took the lead in introducing the DRG system which places hospitals treating Medicare patients on a prospective reimbursement system. No longer would they be reimbursed on the basis of their charges or costs. And the condition of the Medicare Trust Fund with its large prospective deficit makes it almost certain that by 1985 the Congress will have to confront the terms under which the elderly and the disabled will be able to obtain health care in the future.

Although the major shift toward a larger role for the public sector has been centered on the expanded activities of the federal government, we cannot ignore the fact that some states, including such important ones as Massachusetts, New York, and California have insisted on determining the conditions under which hospital care is provided and the conditions under which hospitals are reimbursed. In New York where state controls have been in effect the longest and where state authorities have kept a tight rein on hospital insurance premiums, many of the largest and most prestigious teaching institutions survived only by making major inroads into endowment income and delaying remodeling and rehabilitation of their aging facilities.

Although health insurance providers, both nonprofit and commercial, enjoyed an explosive growth during the last third of a century they neither sought nor obtained significant leverage on the decision-making mechanism. They were satisfied to act as intermediaries negotiating new and improved contracts and paying bills for customers or Medicare patients. It is surprising however that neither business nor labor ever pressured the insurance providers to become more aggressive in controlling provider costs and that the payers in turn did not until quite recently seek to do so themselves.

Part of the explanation lies in the fact that until recently health benefit costs did not loom sufficiently large in the expenditures of major corporations to attract the attention of top management and their benefits staffs. And even now when these cost pressures are such that they warrant attention and business coalitions have organized to facilitate cooperative action among members of the business community at every level, national, state, and local, we still do not know whether payers will be able to exercise leverage over providers. Health care is a highly pluralistic system in which many independent providers operate under different state laws while the federal government finances almost one-third of the total national medical enterprise.

In looking at the recent past before looking ahead we need to take account of only one more new development—the role of private capital and private entrepreneurship in stimulating the recent growth of the health care sector. The last fifteen years have witnessed two major breakthroughs: the nonprofit hospital system has gone to the private capital markets to borrow large sums for construction, rehabilitation, and equipment. And new for-profit hospital and related health care enterprises have gone to the equity markets to obtain much of the capital they need to establish niches in the constantly expanding delivery system from hospital care to HMOs and home care.

The impact of these two developments has already been significant and may by century's end be profound. The independence of the community hospital is reduced when it must meet large interest payments and in the likely event that interest rates remain high its freedom of action will be further reduced. Moreover the increasing presence of aggressive, for-profit hospitals and other health care chains has quickened the environment within which hospitals, physicians, and physician groups must attract and retain patients in order to prosper.

Wall Street and the large for-profit medical enterprises are important new actors on the health care scene and the odds favor their further growth and greater influence on reshaping the system. The formation of large nonprofit hospital systems which is proceeding apace and which is likely in the years ahead to lead to a substantial shrinkage in the number of freestanding institutions must be seen as one response to the challenge of the for-profit system. The restructuring of many nonprofit hospitals to facilitate their vertical integration can also be traced to initiatives that have come from the for-profit sector.

The foregoing account suggests that beneath the largely unchanged health care delivery system which continues to be dominated by fee-for-service practice, physician control has been eroding. New powers are being exercised by both federal and state governments; by the belated but nonetheless heightened interests and concerns of payers to exercise some constraining influences over their steeply rising costs; and by the capital markets and for-profit enterprises. As a concomitant and consequent result of the foregoing, the AMA can no longer determine the direction of public policy.

Based on the transformations which have taken place during the last third of a century we can suggest with some assurance that the shift in power away from physicians and their organizations to government and other payers is likely to continue since government has assumed the responsibility for financing medical care for such a large segment of the population, a responsibility from which it cannot withdraw, and since there is every likelihood that medical care costs will continue to rise, payers will be more, not less, active in seeking to moderate them.

What about the attitudes and behavior of the citizen-patient who in the first and last instance will largely determine both how the private and the public segments of the health care marketplace will be permitted to operate? There is every reason to believe that the strong impetus for the expansion of the system based on the consumer-public interest in broad access for all to quality care will continue. According to recent opinion surveys, the American public generally approves of its health care system although it is concerned about its costliness. Congruent with its widespread diminished respect for all leadership groups from the President to corporate and trade union executives, the public holds physicians in less esteem than in the past although physicians still command substantial respect.

The combination of a significantly higher level of education and greater access to all forms of communications which has characterized the American people has gone far to strip some of the mystique from the practice of medicine and therefore from the power and influence of the physician. Once lost, mystique cannot be readily regained. For better or worse physicians will have to deal with a patient population which will be less and less inclined to follow their orders uncritically.

The combination of more government involvement, more pressures to contain cost, more entrepreneurship aimed at turning health care into a profitable business, and a more skeptical public suggests that American medicine may not be able to attract as high a proportion of the nation's talent as it did in its heyday when young people with a pull towards a medical career realized that they could write their own ticket as practitioner, specialist, academician, researcher. That is no longer the case and is even less likely to obtain by century's end.

The continued erosion of the power and influence of the physician is unlikely to be arrested. What remains unclear is how the redistribution of that power among physicians, government officials, payers, and institutional providers, both large and small, will be worked out. There is no possibility of patients' receiving a desirable level of care unless physicians find their working environments stimulating and professionally rewarding. But this environment will inevitably be constrained by societal needs and financial realities. The challenge that the American people face is to make room for the latter without undermining the former. To reduce the power that physicians have exercised is relatively easy to accomplish now that the competing centers are in place. But to assure that patients continue to receive quality care in a world of shared power is a challenge that neither the United States nor any other advanced nation has yet achieved. It is a worthy challenge for the largest, richest and also one of the oldest of democracies.

Notes

CHAPTER 1

1. British economist A.J. Culyer dates the origins of medical economics as a discipline to the meeting (which I arranged and chaired) of the American Economic Association in Chicago in 1950. See J. van der Gaag and M. Perlman, eds., *Health, Economics, and Health Economics* (New York: Elsevier Science Publishing Co., 1981). In my "Perspectives on the Economics of Medical Care," *American Economic Review* 61, no. 2 (May 1951), I referred to my opening comments at that meeting, to which I appended the comment "some economists do not change their views, at least not very much." The invitation to deliver the Michael M. Davis Lecture was extended to me by Odin Anderson in a phone call while I was reading about Davis in James J. Jones, *Bad Blood: The Tuskegee Experiment* (New York: Free Press, 1981), which to a less skeptical person might point to powers of ESP.

2. E. Ginzberg, "Is Graduate Medical Education Meeting the Country's Needs?" *Bulletin of the New York Academy of Medicine* 50(1199–1203); and E. Ginzberg, "Who Should Pay for Graduate Surgical Education: The Economics of Residency Training," *Surgery* 70(500–502).

3. See E. Ginzberg, E. Brann, D. Hiestand, and M. Ostow, "The Expanding Physician Supply and Health Policy: The Clouded Outlook," *Milbank Memorial Fund Quarterly/Health and Society* 59(508–541); and E. Ginzberg, "The Future Supply of Physicians: From Pluralism to Policy," *Health Affairs* 1(6–19).

4. E. Ginzberg, *A Pattern for Hospital Care: Final Report of the New York State Hospital Study* (New York: Columbia University Press, 1949).

5. E. Ginzberg, "Stockman's Medical Marketplace Reexamined," Letters Section, *Health Affairs* 1(118–120).

6. A. Smith, *An Inquiry into the Nature and Causes of the Wealth of Nations* (1776) (Homewood, Ill: Irwin Press, 1963).

7. R.A. Kessel, "Price Discrimination in Medicine," *Journal of Law and Economics* 1(20–54)

8. M. Feldstein, *Hospital Costs and Health Insurance* (Cambridge: Harvard University Press, 1981).

9. See E. Ginzberg, "Cost Containment—Imaginary and Real," *New England Journal of Medicine* 301(1220–1224); "Competition in Health Care: A Second Opinion," *Hospitals* 56(81–85); "The Grand Illusion of Competition in Health Care," *Journal of the American Medical Association* 249(1857–1859); "Health Institutions and Market Incentives," *Bulletin of the New York Academy of Medicine* 58(545–555); "Health Care Forecast: Adapt to Changing Environment," *Hospital Progress* 63(8–12); "Human Resources as Regulators," *The New Regulators,* A Report of the Ross Health Administration Forum, September 23–25, 1982; "Reforming the Health Care System—Potential and Limits," *Proceedings,* Conference on Demand for Health Care Services sponsored by the Blue Cross and Blue Shield Associations,

April 6–7, 1982, Rosemont, Ill., pp. 27–48; and "Patient Charges, Reimbursements, and Health Care Costs," *Proceedings,* Council of Medical Specialty Societies Invitational Conference to Examine the Roles, Relationships and Issues of Physician and Non-Physician Health Care Providers, October 26–27, 1982, Chicago, pp. 34–40.

10. A.C. Enthoven, *Health Plan: The Only Practical Solution to the Soaring Cost of Medical Care* (Reading, Ma.: Addison-Wesley, 1980).

11. E. Ginzberg, "Services, Health Services, and the General Welfare," in W.J. McNerney, ed., *Working for a Healthier America* (Cambridge: Ballinger, 1980).

12. D.S. Hirshfield, *The Lost Reform* (Cambridge: Harvard University Press, 1970).

13. E. Ginzberg, "Cost Containment—Imaginary and Real," *New England Journal of Medicine* 301(1220–1224).

14. E. Ginzberg, "More Care Is Not Always Better Care," *Inquiry* 19(187–189).

15. A.R. Tarlov, "Shattuck Lecture—The Increasing Supply of Physicians, the Changing Structure of the Health-Services System, and the Future Practice of Medicine," *New England Journal of Medicine* 301(1235–1244).

16. F.C. Moore, "A Community-Size Model for Physician Distribution in the United States: I," *Journal of Clinical Surgery* 1(162–173); and "A Community-Size Model for Physician Distribution in the United States: II," *Journal of Clinical Surgery* 1(242–255).

17. W.J. McNerney, "Health Care Coalitions: New Substance or More Cosmetics?", Michael M. Davis Lecture Seies, Center for Health Administration Studies, Graduate School of Business, University of Chicago, 1982.

18. P.B. Ginsburg and M.J. Curtis, "Prospects for Medicare's Hospital Insurance Trust Fund," Datawatch section, *Health Affairs* 2(102–112).

19. J.M. Clark, *The Social Control of Business,* 2nd ed. (Fairfield, N.J.: Augustus M. Kelley, 1939).

CHAPTER 2

1. A.S. Relman, "The New Medical-Industrial Complex," *New England Journal of Medicine* 303(963–70); "For Physicians, Is It the Lady or the Tiger?" *Internist* 23(10–1); and "The Future of Medical Practice," *Health Affairs* 2(5–19); and J.K. Iglehart, "The Changing World of Private Foundations: An Interview with Dr. David E. Rogers," *Health Affairs* 2(5–22).

2. E. Ginzberg, *A Pattern for Hospital Care: Final Report of the New York State Hospital Study* (New York: Columbia University Press, 1949).

3. R.M. Gibson, "National Health Expenditures, 1978," *Health Care Finance Review* 1(1–36).

4. E. Ginzberg and the Conservation of Human Resources Staff, *Urban Health Services: The Case of New York* (New York: Columbia University Press, 1971), 96–118.

5. R.M. Gibson, D.R. Waldo, and K.R. Levit, "National Health Expenditures, 1982," *Health Care Finance Review* 5(1–31).

6. A.S. Relman, "The Future of Medical Practice," *Health Affairs* 2(5–19).

7. E. Ginzberg, "The Grand Illusion of Competition in Health Care," *Journal of the American Medical Association* 249(1857–1859).

8. D. Wegmiller, "Financing Strategies for Nonprofit Hospital Systems," *Health Affairs* 2(48–54).

9. R. Heyssel, "Commercial Stress and the Academic Medical Center," presented at the annual meeting of the Association of American Medical Colleges, Washington, D.C., November 3, 1981.

10. *Planning Study Report: A Consortium for Assessing Medical Technology* (Washington, D.C.: National Academy Press, Institute of Medicine, National Academy of Sciences, November 1983).

11. A.S. Relman, "Investor owned Hospitals and Health-care Costs," *New England Journal of Medicine* 309(370–372).

12. F.A. Sloan and R.A. Vraciu, "Investor-owned and Not-for-profits Hospitals: Addressing Some Issues," *Health Affairs* 2(25–37); and M.D. Bromberg, "The Medical-Industrial Complex: Our National Defense," *New England Journal of Medicine* 309(1314–1315).

CHAPTER 3

1. R. Reinhold, "Majority in Survey on Health Care Are Open to Changes to Cut Costs," *New York Times,* March 29, 1982:A1(col. 3).

2. H. Waitzkin, "A Marxist View of Medical Care," *Annals of Internal Medicine* 89(264–278); and D.A. Stockman, "Premises for a Medical Marketplace: A Neoconservative's Vision of How to Transform the Health System," *Health Affairs* 1(5–18).

3. K. Davis, *National Health Insurance: Benefits, Costs, and Consequences* (Washington, D.C.: The Brookings Institution, 1975), 9–11.

4. J.A. Califano, Jr., *Governing America: An Insider's Report from the White House and the Cabinet* (New York: Simon & Schuster, 1981), 16–71.

5. J.K. Iglehart, "The New Era of Prospective Payment for Hospitals," *New England Journal of Medicine* 307(1288–1292).

6. C.L. Rosenberg, "Payment by Diagnosis: How the Great Experiment Is Going," *Medical Economics* 59(245–257).

7. D. Banta, "Computed Tomography: Cost Containment Misdirected," *American Journal of Public Health* 70(215–216).

8. M. Feldstein, *Hospital Costs and Health Insurance* (Cambridge: Harvard University Press, 1981).

9. A.C. Enthoven, *Health Plan: The Only Practical Solution to the Soaring Cost of Medical Care* (Reading, Ma.: Addison-Wesley, 1980).

10. J.P. Newhouse, W.G. Manning, C.N. Morris, et al., "Some Interim Results from a Controlled Trial of Cost Sharing in Health Insurance," *New England Journal of Medicine* 305(1501–1507).

11. R. Fein, "Effects of Cost Sharing in Health Insurance: A Call for Caution," *New England Journal of Medicine* 305(1526–1528).

12. C.R. Fisher, "Differences by Age Groups in Health Care Spending," *Health Care Finance Review* 1(65–90).

13. W.A. Glaser, *Paying the Hospital: Foreign Lessons for the United States* (New York: Columbia University Center for the Social Sciences, 1982).

14. H.S. Luft, "How Do Health-Maintenance Organizations Achieve Their 'Savings'?" Rhetoric and Evidence," *New England Journal of Medicine* 298(1336–1343).

15. L.D. Brown, "Competition and Health Cost Containment: Cautions and Conjectures," *Milbank Memorial Fund Quarterly/Health and Society* 59(145–189).

16. M. Lalonde, *A New Perspective on the Health of Canadians: A Working Document* (Ottawa: Information Canada, 1975), 506.

17. European Coronary Surgery Study Group, "Prospective Randomised Study of Coronary Artery Bypass Surgery in Stable Angina Pectoris: Second Interim Report," *Lancet* 2(491–495).

18. J.K. Iglehart, "Funding the End-Stage Renal-Disease Program," *New England Journal of Medicine* 306(492–496).

19. M. Friedman, *Capitalism and Freedom* (Chicago: Phoenix Books, 1962), 149–160.

20. E. Ginzberg and A.M. Yohalem, eds., *The University Medical Center and the Metropolis* (New York: Josiah Macy, Jr. Foundation, 1974).

21. L.E. Demkovich, "Will Medicare for Hospice Programs Cut Costs or Become a Boondoggle?" *National Journal* 141(1639–1641).

22. *Third Report to the President and Congress on the Status of Health Professions Personnel in the United States* (Rockville, Md.: Department of Health and Human Services, 1982). VI-7.

23. E. Ginzberg, "The Future Supply of Physicians: From Pluralism to Policy," *Health Affairs* 1(6–19).

24. *Healthy People: The Surgeon General's Report on Health Promotion and Disease Prevention* (Washington, D.C.: Department of Health, Education, and Welfare, 1979), vii–x.

CHAPTER 5

1. A.C. Enthoven, "Consumer-Choice Health Plan," *New England Journal of Medicine* 298(650–658,709–720).

2. *S. 1968, Health Incentives Reform Act of 1979,* introduced by Senator Durenberger (R.-Minn.) on November 1, 1979; *H.R. 5740, The Health Care Cost Restraint Act of 1979,* introduced by Representative Ullman (D.-Oreg.) on October 30, 1979; and *H.R. 7527, The National Health Care Reform Act,* introduced by Representatives Gephardt (D.-Mo.) and Stockman (R.-Mich.) on June 9, 1980.

3. M. Freeland, G. Calat, and C.E. Schendler, "Projections of National Health Expenditures, 1980, 1985, and 1990," *Health Care Finance Review* 1(9).

4. For the tax benefits, see Congressional Budget Office, *Tax Subsidies for Medical Care: Current Policies and Possible Alternatives* (Washington, D.C.: GPO, January 1980), xi.

5. E. Ginzberg, "Services, Health Services, and the General Welfare," in W.J. McNerney, ed., *Working for a Healthier America* (Cambridge: Ballinger, 1980).

6. L.A. Aday, R. Andersen, and G.V. Fleming, *Health Care in the U.S.: Equitable for Whom?* (Beverly Hills: Sage, 1980), 148.

7. R.M. Gibson, "National Health Expenditures, 1979," *Health Care Finance Review* 2(1–36).

8. M.S. Carroll, "Private Health Insurance Plans in 1976: An Evaluation," *Social Security Bulletin* 41(3–16).

9. *Controlling the Supply of Hospital Beds* (Washington, D.C.: Institute of Medicine, 1976).

10. R.M. Hendrickson, "Hard Times Ahead for Physicians?" *American Medical News* 23(1–3).

11. Association of American Medical Colleges, Testimony on S. 1968, The Health Incentives Reform Act, submitted to the Subcommittee on Health, Committee on Finance, U.S. Senate, March 18, 1980.

CHAPTER 6

1. A.C. Enthoven, *Health Plan: The Only Practical Solution to the Soaring Cost of Medical Care* (Reading, Ma.: Addison-Wesley, 1980).

2. Health Insurance Institute, *Competition in the Health Care System* (Washington, D.C.: Health Insurance Institute, 1981).

3. A.C. Enthoven, *Health Plan: the Only Practical Solution to the Soaring Cost of Medical Care* (Reading, Ma.: Addison-Wesley, 1980).

4. M. Feldstein, *Hospital Costs and Health Insurance* (Cambridge: Harvard University Press, 1981).

5. Blue Cross and Blue Shield Associations, *Competition and Consumer Choice—A Third Party Payer's Perspective—Medicare Vouchers* (Washington, D.C.: Blue Cross, 1981).

6. W. McClure, "Structure and Incentive Problems in Economic Regulation of Medical Care," *Milbank Memorial Fund Quarterly/Health and Society* 59 (107–144).

7. L. Brown, *Prepaid Medical Groups and Public Policy* (Washington, D.C.: The Brookings Institution, 1982).

8. K.J. Arrow, "Uncertainty and the Welfare Economics of Medical Care," *American Economic Review* 53(941–973).

9. J.P. Newhouse, W.G. Manning, C.N. Morris, et al., *Some Interim Results from a Controlled Trial of Cost Sharing in Health Insurance* (Santa Monica: The Rand Corporation, 1982).

10. Congressional Budget Office, *Health Planning: Issues for Reauthorization* (Washington, D.C.: GPO, 1982).

CHAPTER 7

1. U.S. *Economic Report of the President* (Washington, D.C.: GPO, 1982), p. 150.
2. *Ibid.*
3. E. Ginzberg, "Competition and Cost Containment," *New England Journal of Medicine* 303(1112–1115).
4. E. Ginzberg, "The Many Faces of Competition in Health Care," *Hospital Practice* 16(13–14).
5. E. Ginzberg, "Competition in Health Care: A Second Opinion," *Hospitals* 56(81–85).

CHAPTER 11

1. E. Moses and A. Roth, "Nursepower: What Do Statistics Reveal About the Nation's Nurses?," *American Journal of Nursing* 79(1745–1756).
2. M.A. Wandelt, P.M. Pierce, and R.R. Widdowson, "Why Nurses Leave Nursing and What Can Be Done About It," *American Journal of Nursing* 81(72–77).
3. C.S. Weisman, "Recruitment and Retention of Hospital Nurses in the 1980s," presented at the meeting of the National Association of Nurse Recruiters, Philadelphia, Pa., July 31, 1981.
4. E. Moses and A. Roth, "Nursepower: What Do Statistics Reveal About the Nation's Nurses?" *American Journal of Nursing* 79(1745–1756).
5. E. Ginzberg, *A Program for the Nursing Profession* (New York: Macmillan, 1948).
6. J. Ulsafer-Van Lanen, "Lateral Promotion Keeps Skilled Nurses in Direct Patient Care," *Hospitals* 55(87–90).
7. R.E. Weiss, G. Sobiech, and J.E. Sauer, "Innovative Plan Solves Nurse Shortage Problem," *Hospitals* 55(78–84).

CHAPTER 12

1. U.S. Department of Health, Education, and Welfare, Bureau of Health Manpower, *A Report on Allied Health Manpower,* prepared for the Committee on Interstate and Foreign Commerce, House of Representatives, and the Committee on Labor and Human Resources, Senate (Washington, D.C.: GPO, November 16, 1979).
2. U.S. Departments of Labor and Health, Education, and Welfare, *Health Careers Guidebook,* 4th ed (Washington, D.C.: GPO, 1979).
3. *Ibid.,* p. 137.
4. U.S. Department of Health, Education, and Welfare, Bureau of Health Manpower, *A Report on Allied Health Manpower,* prepared for the Committee on Interstate and Foreign Commerce, House of Representatives, and the Committee on Labor and Human Resources, Senate (Washington, D.C.: GPO, November 16, 1979), pp. 1–7.
5. M. Roemer and R. Roemer, *Health Manpower Policies Under Five National Health Care Systems* (Washington, D.C.: GPO, 1978), p. 55.
6. *Ibid.,* pp. 36, 56.
7. U.S. Department of Health, Education, and Welfare, Bureau of Health Manpower, *A Report on Allied Health Manpower,* prepared for the Committee on Interstate and Foreign Commerce, House of Representatives, and the Committee on Labor and Human Resources, Senate (Washington, D.C.: GPO, November 16, 1979), p. 50.

CHAPTER 13

1. Correspondence, *New England Journal of Medicine* 262(367).
2. L.H. Aiken, C.E. Lewis, J. Craig, et al., "The Contribution of Specialists to the Delivery of Primary Care: A New Perspective," *New England Journal of Medicine* 300(1363).
3. H. Wise, "Health Manpower Training: The Team Approach," in E. Ginzberg and A.M. Yohalem, eds., *The University Medical Center and the Metropolis* (New York: Josiah Macy, Jr. Foundation, 1974).

CHAPTER 14

1. *Statistical Abstract of the United States, 1957* (Washington, D.C.: GPO, 1957).

2. J.R. Krevans, "Transformation of Medicine Since 1945," *Journal of Medical Education* 59(75–78).

3. R.G. Petersdorf, "Managing the Revolution of Medical Care," *Journal of Medical Education* 59(79–90).

4. *Statistical Abstract of the United States, 1982–1983* (Washington, D.C.: GPO, 1982).

5. Association of American Medical Colleges, *Medical Research—Maintaining America's Preeminence* (Washington, D.C.: The Association, 1983).

6. C.M. Taeuber, *America in Transition: An Aging Society* (Washington, D.C.: GPO, 1983).

7. R.G. Petersdorf, "Is the Establishment Defensible?" *New England Journal of Medicine* 309(1053–1057).

8. Subcommittee on Health of the Committee on Ways and Means, U.S. House of Representatives, *Conference on the Future of Medicare* (Washington, D.C.: GPO, 1983).

9. B.B. Roe, "The UCR Boondoggle: A Death Knell for Private Practice?," *New England Journal of Medicine* 305(41–45).

CHAPTER 16

1. Department of Health and Human Services, *Health: United States, 1980* (Hyattsville, Md.: GPO, 1980), p. 220. The figures have been adjusted for inflation.

2. Henry J. Aaron and William B. Schwartz, *The Painful Prescription: Rationing Health Care* (Washington, D.C.: Brookings Institution, 1984).

Index